where'd i put my boobs?

where'd i put my boobs?

Life Goes on During Breast Cancer

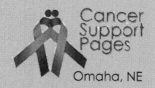

Cancer
Support
Pages

Omaha, NE

SARAH BALL

Paperback ISBN: 978-0-9848175-1-1
LCCN: 2012930045

Printed in United States
10 9 8 7 6 5 4 3 2 1

Contents

Introduction

Living the life of a Navy brat and Air Force wife, I developed a grit, an independence, that is unique to the lifestyle of the military. I was used to moves, fixing things myself, deployments (military business trips), and being alone.

Our sons, Fred, sixteen, and Alex, fourteen, are used to the temporary single-parent household during deployments. Among other coping skills in a military environment, we learned to speak in acronyms and tell time on a twenty-four-hour schedule where 1700 hours is 5:00 p.m.

Living the life of a two-time cancer veteran (breast, and later ovarian), I developed a similar grit. I got used to appointments, procedures, treatments, and surgeries. I learned to live with pain, fear, and the possibility of recurrence. I learned medical terminology and how to interpret the test results.

I had been surrounded by breast cancer since my mom got it when I was a little girl, and she was in her mid-thirties. She has had it more than once, gone through the chemotherapy and the radiation. She made it out the other side.

My aunts, her sisters, both had breast cancer. They were also young and made it out the other side.

My older brother had skin cancer at twenty-two. He also made it out the other side.

I live in a family of survivors—of cancer veterans.

All of them were young when diagnosed, all of them survived. I live in a family of survivors— of cancer veterans. It was never a question that I would get it. It was also not a question that if I was careful and took care of myself that I would beat it as well. It was just an expectation. So when I got tested for the gene, it was only a formality. I knew I had the BRCA2 gene. I knew I would get breast cancer.

The genetic BRCA cancers are tripped off by estrogen. The theory right now is that if you get rid of the estrogen, you can reduce your risks so much that you may not get cancer at all. I liked this idea. I was done with my pregnancy years, and I was much more willing to be menopausal than a cancer patient. After much deliberation, I decided to have my ovaries removed before I got breast cancer as a way to hopefully add some validity to that type of treatment. My surgery was scheduled, and I was ordered to have my routine mammogram that was due before the surgery.

Guess what we found?

I began to write a daily Facebook posting as a way to tell my friends and family how I was doing after I was diagnosed with stage I breast cancer. I had been through some other traumatic things in my life recently that had left me feeling very much alone. As it turns out I only felt alone because no one knew quite what to say.

When the diagnosis came in that I had breast cancer, I was suddenly surrounded by people who loved me, cared about me, and wanted to help me on this journey with their support. This was something they knew they could do for me. I was flooded with phone calls, emails, letters, and flowers, and I could not keep up with it all. It was wonderful.

Although I loved the calls, I spent something like six hours a day on the phone for the first couple of days after diagnosis with everyone wanting to see how I was taking the news. I decided to do some journaling on my Facebook page as an easy way for people to know how I was and what I was going through.

After diagnosis, very often the true strength of a marriage becomes clear. Many marriages either end during this time, or they strengthen. In my case, it evolved right under my nose, and I didn't even realize it.

Things between Lee and me had been very bad for a long time. We had been hanging on by a thread. We had lost a daughter, and part of me blamed him, because he was not there for me like I needed him to be. Our marriage had been rocky from the start because of the typical mistakes people make in marriages. The problem was that I saw them as fatal flaws, not as normal mistakes in a marriage between two imperfect people.

We were in a very dark, unfriendly place when I was diagnosed, but gradually, grudgingly, we evolved into a place of safety and peace that was still admittedly shaky, but a very different place than we had ever been. I have to say, it was a good place, and I almost missed it because I was so busy being angry about the past that I was ignoring my present. It took many stories that I heard from many cancer veterans to finally get it through my head that I was the one being stubborn, stupid, and blind—not to mention unforgiving.

I need to begin in December 2009. The wedding ring had been removed and was sitting in a drawer.   My husband, Lee, an Air Force officer, was in Baghdad, Iraq, two months into a six-month military deployment. Things between us had deteriorated to the point that when he left in October, I had already decided I wanted a divorce. I didn't feel it was right to spring that on him then, so I waited, planning on telling him upon his return. My story begins there.

If you are reading this because you have cancer, first I say to you: Welcome to the club with the most members who never wanted to be included! Next, I say: You are a warrior and a veteran, fighting for your life. What are you going to do next?

I find that people with a cancer diagnosis either seem to wake up and get moving, or decide to slow down. Either way, you re-evaluate your life and decide what is worth living for. That part of the journey is wonderful,

Welcome to the club with the most members who never wanted to be included!

and fascinating, and very surprising. Think of the cancer as your version of a cocoon. You are a fuzzy caterpillar. Cancer wraps you in a cocoon, and after treatment, you find yourself morphed into an amazing butterfly. You'll be beautiful in ways you never ever dreamed, and with a brand new pair of wings to fly.

Do not be disheartened during your isolation in the cocoon. You are not as alone as you feel. Allow others to reach for you and hold them tight. Have faith that God will make it all work out for His will in the end, and let that be enough.

Join me now on my journey. I hope it inspires you, and most of all, I pray your butterfly days ahead will be filled with a new joy.

Tough Stuff

I lost a daughter.

Well, I was losing a daughter. It's a long, horrible, terribly sad story, beginning with a Russian orphanage. As has been in the news recently, and off and on over the years, these kids have issues. Some children more than others. No one knows exactly what happens to these kids in the orphanages from a mental standpoint. Some kids do fine when adopted. They adapt, and they are able to trust again, and love, and be all right. Some kids are not so resilient. Some kids never recover from the horrors of what they lived.

The orphanages try their best to take good care of the kids, but no matter how hard they try, the kids are neglected out of sheer numbers. They are abused sexually by other kids, and many times also by adults. They are physically abused or had wounds left untreated due to lack of supervision or lack of medical supplies. Food choices are limited, as well as amounts, so they often suffered from malnutrition. They are neglected on every level. Antibiotics are scarce, so the kids are all sick for prolonged periods of time, and often have parasites from contaminated drinking water and living conditions. They lose trust; they take on a warped, unsafe view of the world where they are in a feral survival-instinct state out of necessity.

When they are adopted, many of them are able to move on, but others are not. Others stay in that feral, survival state. Depending on the severity of the issues, the only one to see the child as they really are is the adoptive mother. I believe this is a combination of her being the main caretaker, and almost an instinctual need to blame their real mothers for abandoning them. It's so different for each child, for each orphanage. But mark my words, I knew better than most. I had visited several orphanages over the course of a few weeks, in different years.

I had seen the abandoned children from the perspective of an observer, not just an adoptive parent, taking information about a child back to a potential adoptive family. I had interacted with the children as a group, I had seen some of what happens to them when no one was looking, which was often.

With staying in this state of mistrust, and anger, and survival, these kids develop all sorts of nasty, scary mental illnesses. They were very real, and the kids do not just get better if you hug them more, feed them regularly, get them counseling, or give them medication. These kids, just like anyone with any mental illness, only get better if they choose to. The difficult thing with these children is that they trust no one, and often choose not to get better, especially if they feel they can become successful in punishing the mom or creating their own version of a "safe world" that works for them alone.

They were abused kids who become abusers. They abuse from very early on, just as they were. Because of the damage to these feral kids, regular therapy does not work for most of them. If they are not reached as they grow, they become smarter, and stronger, and more manipulative; they could become a danger to others. They start to hurt and abuse others, starting with the adoptive mother. They plot to kill, and start practicing on animals and on those smaller and weaker than themselves.

In 2008, at the age of six, my daughter, who was plucked from a Russian orphanage in 2000, pretended to be mentally retarded because she realized that people let her do things that otherwise would be considered inappropriate. Things like pretending to not be able to button her pants to get people (especially her teachers) to put their hands in her pants to button them. Then she would come home and tell me the teachers put their hands down her pants. Eventually things progressed to the point of her trying to sexually abuse other children; she was hurting animals, trying to kill more than one cat, and she did kill a parrot.

I took her to therapy since the day we got her home, but unfortunately, not everyone who claims to be qualified to reach these kids actually is. I endured years of abuse by her. Physical: she was always hitting and kicking, and trying to bite me. She would purposefully break things that were within reach, it didn't matter whose it was or what it was. Nothing had value to her.

Emotionally: She screamed at me for several hours each day, telling me how horrible I was, how worthless, how I stole her from her mother in Russia to be her slave. Mentally: She was the sweetest thing to everyone else around until the very end of her time with us, so when I told people what was happening, they didn't believe me. Some still don't. Her levels of manipulation were astounding—and frightening.

I was accused of not letting her have friends, but I could see her trying to sexually abuse the other children. I was told to quit pushing her so hard, that she was delayed, yet when put in positions where proving herself was to her benefit, she proved more intelligent than the other children. She abused me, and I was told to "be nicer" by people who had never been in my home, and had never seen her act up with me. I researched, I talked to nationally renowned specialists, I went to seminars, and I tried everything I could.

By the time I finally found someone who could help her, she was becoming too difficult to handle, and dangerous. When she told me that she wanted to kill me and her brother, as well as how she would do it, and that she fanaticized having sex with her father and other brother, I could take it no more. I could not keep everyone safe from her.

She needed serious help that I could not provide.

We looked into places that were qualified to help her, but insurance would not cover the $1,000 a week. We found a residential treatment center that knew what they were doing in Denver, but insurance would only pay for her for five months, and she would not have been ready to come home by then, nor would I be ready for her. I had to keep everyone safe all the time. I simply could not do it anymore.

She had done a six-month in-home respite care with one of the best-trained caretakers in the area, and even the caretaker could not keep my daughter from hurting others. I had to give her over to the state and pray that they would get her treatment, and in doing so, I had to give up being her mom. She wanted that, and told me so happily.

We had her psychologically evaluated before this decision was made, and the results were flat out scary. Had she had the same test results as an adult, she would be considered to have the mental profile of a serial killer.

No kidding.

The doctor who did the testing thanked me for holding out so long and trying my best.

All the people who knew these kids and what they were capable of agreed that I did an awesome job, but that it just wasn't enough. When the state first got her, they were calling me for resources to help her. Because all of the agencies qualified to deal with her were out of state, however, she was put someplace local.

I did love her. I tried to prove that to her. I did everything I could, tried everything, not always successfully. But in the end it didn't matter. She chose to leave. She chose to behave in such a way that we could not keep her. She was always in control of her own behavior, which made that reality scarier. She never asked for any of her things, none of her toys, nothing. She was told she could have them, and she didn't want them. She didn't want us. She didn't want me.

The state still had everything tied up in court, so things were not over yet. I had been so devastated by things that I could not even look at girl clothes or toys without wanting to cry and run away, even though she had been out of our house, and I had been safe from her, for two years. I felt like they had not listened to a word I said about what she did and the state shuffled her around several times, so did not exhibit any of the ugly behaviors at all.

She has since remained in a "honeymoon" period of behavior. They allowed her to get worse, by not pressing her to get better. That was my opinion. I've been badly hurt by her, and the emotional scars were terrible. Some days I wish they were visible to show to those who did not believe me. There were those within the state who did try very hard to help her, and even they were ignored.

Was I seeing a counselor? No. Why? Because the one I was seeing when everything came to a head with my daughter asked me the following question: "How does it feel to throw your daughter away like the trash?"

Yes, a therapist asked me that.

I was so devastated, that I have not trusted a therapist enough to go to one. I did see my pastor, but that was it. With my faith, and my friends, and the family who has stood by me, it was enough.

Losing a child is the worst thing in the world, and it doesn't matter how you lose them. Losing them in such a way that you cannot openly grieve is worse still.

Wife of the Year Award

I can't believe what I just did. I can't believe that I could do that to someone, even as mad as I was. Lee was in Iraq. Baghdad. He was getting shelled, hearing gun fire, explosions, he was far from home, and what do I do? I blurt out that I wanted a divorce while we were talking via Skype. I didn't want to do that. I didn't want to tell him this way. I was angry because we were having yet another argument, but that did not make it OK.

I felt horrible, and guilty. I admit that part of me felt justified and more resolved on my course of action. But I still felt like a horrible person for what I had done. It was not OK to put that kind of stress on a man when he was in a war like that. Part of their psyche hangs on to good things by thinking about what they have to look forward to when they return home. I had stolen that peace from him. Even if it was a false dream for him, and I knew that, it was real for him, and I destroyed that.

I now worried about how he would cope over there knowing that coming home would result in my leaving. Many guys in war-time situations when faced with news like that often snap and commit suicide or all sorts of other possible ugly scenarios associated with traumatic stress. How I could I do that? How could I let my tongue slip in that fashion? How could I be so selfish?

This ranks as my top worst moment as a human being on this earth. What an honor.

Oophorectomies

On the 27th of January 2010 I was scheduled to get a salpingo-oophorectomy. I was going to get my ovaries and fallopian tubes removed. At that time I scheduled the surgery, I did not have cancer, but was probably going to. All the women on my mom's side older than I, with only two exceptions (one of mom's cousins and her daughter), had had breast cancer. There was never a doubt in my mind I would get it, but I was not worried, because I knew to look, to watch, to get the mammograms, etc. So when the genetic test came back positive, it was of no surprise at all. The BRCA2 gene was responsible for three cancers: breast, ovarian, and skin cancer. We had skin cancer in our family too. My brother was unlucky enough to get that bugger in his early twenties, but my mom has had it too.

So I found out about the full genetic testing results in the fall of '09. Then it was a matter of deciding what to do about it. My breast cancer doctor recommended prophylactic bilateral mastectomies (fancy terms for having the breasts removed "just in case"). However, my gynecologist suggested complete prophylactic hysterectomy and oophorectomy-removing the ovaries (again, "just in case").

You see, they had discovered that the production of estrogen was what triggers this gene to create cancer. I needed to get rid of the estrogen. The two main estrogen-producing organs of the body were ovaries and the breasts. So we wanted to get those removed. The ovaries were the biggest producers, so it made sense to get rid of those first.

Now, having a complete hysterectomy was huge. Previously, it was major abdominal surgery where you were removing a ton of female organs in the nether regions, and it throws you into immediate menopause for those of us who are not naturally there yet. They now have procedures to do this laparoscopically, which means they don't have to cut you open from one side to the other, but can make a few small holes and pull everything out from there. So recovery isn't as bad as years ago. But it is still a major trauma to the body.

So, with the hysterectomy, they would remove the ovaries, fallopian tubes, uterus (where the baby grows), cervix (where the baby's head has to squeeze through), and neck of the vagina. Now, didn't quote me here, this was just my understanding, but I know I am not too far off. Anyhow, this is what was involved. Well, in my family, we had breast cancer and skin cancer. No one (yet) has ever had ovarian, uterine, or cervical cancers. So, since my doctors disagreed, I got to choose. Lovely.

If you ever want to shock the doctors, especially the specialists who were the leading ones in their fields, tell them you disagree with their recommendations. It's interesting. Not really fun, but when you have to make the choice: get educated! My surgeons were great in their own fields; leading scientists and surgeons who were both on the team that helped discover the link of the BRCA2 gene to estrogen. Well, let's just say they were not used to anyone disagreeing with them. So it seemed to really stop them cold (and not in the best way), that I would not do exactly as they wanted.

When you have to make the choice: get educated!

I had to decide what my risks were to get the best care. I had the best docs, but the decision was in my hands. That was a bit scary. So I had to sit down and reason it all out. My family has the breast cancer first and foremost. That was the number one concern. That would indicate getting the prophylactic mastectomies (I'm getting tired of writing all these huge words. That is why in the medical field, like the military, there are a ton of abbreviations.). However, since the cancer was activated by estrogen production, that alone would reduce the risk dramatically (by like eighty percent) of getting breast cancer.   So I should remove the ovaries. Get the hysterectomy? No. The estrogen was gone without the ovaries. The BRCA2 does not include the increased chance of the other female cancers, aside from breast cancer with the ovaries gone. Getting a Pap smear would detect those cancers, so I could be careful, just in case. Just like getting the mammograms!

I decided to get just the ovaries and fallopian tubes removed. In case you were wondering, the thing with the fallopian tubes was that they retain enough of the estrogen to maintain an amount of risk (think a drinking straw when pulled out of your Pepsi still has soda in it). Therefore, they take the fallopian tubes.

OK, let's do it.

That was scheduled for the twenty seventh of January. It was an outpatient procedure that lasts only an hour, and I'd be up and around to normal activity in a few days. Then I got to deal with menopause. Not gradual menopause, but wholly crud, here it comes, menopause. Fine, we would deal. It was a reasonable enough of a surgery.

I had told Lee that I didn't want him to come home for the ovary removal surgery. I truly did not want him there. It seemed stupid to me to have him struggle to get home in time, a trip that would be fraught with potential delays, and missed connections, spanning several days, only to be home for the surgery and three-day recovery, then turn around and go back. Besides, I had planned on moving out after he got home, but I wasn't ready to make him aware of the plans I was making. I did not want him in the house.

Besides, I thought it was a nice thought to try to be through the majority of the nastiness of menopause (the tough emotional stuff hits hard and fast, but levels off after a few months) before he got home.

Anyhow, before the surgery, it was recommended that I get a mammogram, just in case. I was due anyhow, as I got them every six months now. This time they wanted to do an MRI of the breast. This was not a mammogram. I keep lumping them together because their end result for both procedures was to look for the cancers. The MRI was done with a contrast, which, joy, was done with an IV push.

Crap.

They didn't tell me that. During the procedure the vein in my hand blew, but it didn't bubble up, so we didn't know it had blown. I ended up with painful contrast in my hand (that hurt for a month), and almost none on the resulting MRI. So I was told that the test had to be redone. The MRI was done on the twelfth of January. My radiologist was not notified that this was a pre-surgical thing, so there was no rush on it. She didn't get back to me until the afternoon of Friday the twenty second of January that the test did not go, and we had to repeat it.

Great. Right before my surgery I got to screw around with blowing more veins? Then she let me know that something did show up, and we really needed to look at it since it may affect my surgery. Now, at this point, I was thinking they would be doing, at most, a biopsy during the surgery, OK. No problem. But I asked if we could do the regular mammogram instead, and she said that was fine.

I went in, and we did a regular mammogram.

I love to look at radiographs and ultrasounds and such. I had taken a basic radiology class. I could see a lot of the stuff you otherwise had to be trained to see. I can't tell you what I see, but I see it. So I look at the digital mammograms right after they were taken, and I see it, too. We repeated a mammo on the area. Yup, something's there. So we then did an ultrasound, and yup, it's there.

My radiologist told me that if it was anyone else, they would have missed it, but since it was me (yeah, they knew me ...), they wanted to do a biopsy.

Now.

As I sat there in this little white bathrobe in this cool room, we got everything set up, and waited to get insurance approval.

Now.

The radiologist called the oncologist's office and asked the head nurse to find out if she needed a referral from my insurance to do the biopsy. I waited for three hours, sitting in the little white robe in the waiting area, awaiting the call to either get the biopsy, or go home. I finally went back out to the receptionist, who called the oncologist nurse back.

The response from the head nurse?

"Oh, well it takes about three days to get a referral through." She had not listened to the fact that the biopsy was a rush, nor had she followed up with my insurance to find out what, if anything, needed to be done.

I got on the phone myself, and within five minutes I reached my insurance company and found out that I did not need a referral since the mammogram found something, and I was clear to get the biopsy. I was not a happy camper with the nurse.

OK, whatever, I was not my first biopsy, it was my second. I was not worried, and I knew about what to expect. It would raise your blood pressure, but it didn't hurt and really wasn't uncomfortable. Good thing. The size of the needle was about the size of a large coffee straw, and about 6 inches long. Um, yeah … I really liked lidocaine by this point, and considered buying lots of stock in it.

The radiologist had to cut a small slit on the skin before inserting the big honking needle. Good choice. Then the pushing began. I had no idea how dense breast tissue was, as in, how truly dense breast tissue was. I've done dissection, I figured the density was somewhere between fat and muscle, probably about the density of the liver. The needle would meet some resistance, but not much.

Wrong. It took her thirty minutes of pushing with considerable force to get the needle to the proper spot for the biopsy. Just getting the needle into the lump was quite an experience as she really had to push hard, and suddenly there was this "POP" sound and I could feel a sudden give (but no pain).

Now I was watching the monitor for the ultrasound, which was guiding the radiologist to the lump, so I knew she had not pushed all the way through to the other side of my breast, which was what it felt like. Then a nice noisy suction machine took out the biopsy area, which technically took the entire lump.

She put a rush on the biopsy and got it to pathology immediately. We knew by lunchtime the next day. As a matter of fact, I was on Skype with Lee at about 1330 when the call came in.

Yes, it was cancer.

OK, no biggie. That was truly my first thought. My second was "crap, there goes surgery." See, the other reason I decided to go the route I was planning was the hope that maybe, just maybe, I could keep my breasts after all. Maybe the estrogen reduction due to the ovary removal would be just enough to never get breast cancer. It was a theory. Maybe, just maybe that could be the case for me. Now that theory was shot. No such luck. Crap, I was going to lose the breasts anyhow.

I had to grudgingly admit I was glad I was on the video chat with him when the call came in. But I was still so mad at him I didn't want to admit that, even to myself. That call from my radiologist changed everything.

I knew that what lie ahead of me would not be a simple three-day recovery. I would need help. I didn't want help, but I knew that I could not have cared for the boys, and driven them everywhere they needed, or fixed them dinner, etc. I needed Lee home.

I remember very clearly telling him that I needed him to come home, but that it was not for me. I would not need him to take care of me, but to take care of the boys. He would have to do that since I could not. I didn't want to be put in a position of having to be cared for by him. Yet at the same time, I did not feel right having to expect my friends to pick up the slack that I knew a husband should be providing, such as trips to doctors' appointments, etc. I hated to admit it to myself, and I was not about to admit it to him, but I needed him to care for me.

I had callously told Lee I wanted a divorce while he was sitting in a war zone, and now I had the gall to expect him to take care of me during cancer? How stupid was I? I really was not sure what to expect from him. I would not have blamed him for telling me I was on my own. I would have understood if he told me to get out of the house. It made sense to me that he would refuse to help with what I needed. After all, I was the ex-to-be ... and I had brought this on myself.

Then the question was whether I should have the original surgery tomorrow or not. Again, I called both my surgeons—you know, the ones who keep disagreeing with each other.

And, again, they disagreed.

Well, let's think about this. I would still need both surgeries. The ovary one was fast, simple, with the least possibilities of complications, and I would be healed before my cancer surgery.

However, I now had cancer, and that was the number one priority: GET IT OUT. If I had this "little surgery," and there were any complications, it could delay getting my cancer surgery done. That was not an option. Yet again, I got to tell one of my renowned specialist surgeons that I was going to disagree with him.

Oh, what they must think of me. They could tell I was informed; they just were not used to being disagreed with. I was never normal.

So, here I was. Plans had changed, I would lose my breasts, but I would beat cancer. I would be a veteran, and if I was like the rest of my family, this would not be the end of it, but just the beginning because it would return in some form or another.

That's OK. I would wait, I would be prepared. I kind of felt like I was the jealous father awaiting the inevitable arrival of one of *those* boys at the door for my daughter, so I wait, cleaning my shotgun over and over, and when he arrives, I let him know he is not welcome. He may go away, but another one would eventually come around again, so the shotgun remains at the ready...

I would get the breasts removed in a month or two. Heal from this one first, and then schedule the second to remove my ovaries. And the story would continue.

Blonde and DD's

Cancer would not win, but it would get a piece of me. Now with the reality of the surgery coming up and the following reconstruction, I had certain realities of when it was all over how I would be different. I read a romance novel today, and there were lots of references to certain forms of affection including certain body parts that I would soon be missing. Well, shoot, that's a bit depressing. It's more than the loss of just the breast, but a part of intimacy would be gone as well: intimacy that I would sorely miss. It was something of real significance, and it would be gone. The memories of it would not be enough. Think it's no big deal? Try thinking of your most wonderful, intimate memory, and what that may include. Uh-huh. Thought so.

Yes, I would live; yes, I would beat cancer. That was my silver lining. But I still had to deal with the realities of how it would change my life for forever in a way I would

> Cancer would not win, but it would get a piece of me.

not want. Then I had to turn around and go through menopause. Joy. That was another alteration to intimacy. Lovely. Fine. This sucks. I would prefer to have just caught this earlier (I tried!), and gone through menopause, and kept the breasts. No such luck.

So much for the seventeen credit hours I was taking trying to finish my associate's degree in biology. Dang it! At least I got to keep one online class: nutrition. I've had so many classes I've taken, and so many times I have had to drop out. I'm sick and tired of it. I'm tired of "you could just go back later." When was later? Every time I think it's "later," something else comes up. I knew I was an intelligent individual, but was I still so caught up in the fact that the blonde was natural that I NEED a stupid piece of paper to prove to the world that I actually possessed a brain?

Yeah, like that would work. Maybe I should work on flirting, and playing dumb more, and get the DDs. Still not my style. Too bad, might have been interesting. I wonder if they could just install a zipper so I could change sizes when I decided I need a better fit for a strapless dress. Or when I want to look better in a bikini? I suppose I could ask—maybe cock my head to the side, use the voice of Karen from *Will and Grace* that I do so well, and flutter my eyes. Why do I think that if I did that my plastic surgeon would only look at me and ask me if I wanted a nose job to go with the new pair? It would be a bonus he could throw in for my being a good customer.

Cancer may get a piece of me. Wish I could give cancer a piece of my mind! Hmm, I should be careful what I wish for. I couldn't yell at it. I couldn't tell it where to

27

go. I couldn't discourage it. I couldn't berate it. I couldn't reason with it. It's my body attacking itself. Why? Who the h-e-double-hockey sticks knows? It just was. It's like a miniature war going on inside my body at a cellular level. Cancer cell versus antibody. Goliath versus David. The analogy isn't too far off.

Did you know that cancer cells are huge by comparison to the normal cells surrounding it? Yup, about four times bigger. They are huge. They're easy to spot on the laboratory slide. I wish there lived a little David in each of us capable of slaying that Goliath so we could all be OK, and not have body parts removed.

There are lessons for all of us to learn in each thing we go through. We also have to remember that the lesson isn't always just for us. Letting others help us, letting others love us, letting others care for us was part of the lesson for them and us. I hope I learn it well enough the first time that I don't have to repeat the lesson.

Wanna See My Scars?

I had heard someone who was worried about me say I was a bit too OK with everything. Rest assured, I had not lost it (not that I ever did find it in the first place), nor was I being blind to what this all meant. I had lived with this cloud all my life. It was actually kind of nice to finally deal with it so I could put it behind me instead of always looking over my shoulder for it. The fact was, breast cancer, MY breast cancer, does not scare me. Many of my family members had gone there before, and all of them had come back. I would beat it; of that there was no doubt. Would I be this optimistic if it were any other type of cancer? Probably not. But I was not prepared for any other type of cancer; I was prepared for breast cancer.

I was prepared for breast cancer.

I would admit, however, that the realities of the reconstruction did bother me. Here's a thought: could I be arrested for indecent exposure if I show off my scars? After all, it's not indecent if you were not showing the nipple (ala Janet Jackson here), and if I had any afterward, they would be fake too. So, wanna see my scars?

Right now I think that I would feel as if they were not real, not mine. As if they were some random appendage I now had to carry instead of what was me. Wanna see 'em? Sure, nothing rude about that. They're fake, not real, pretend, tattooed on: NOT ME.

Then again, I was not there yet. Could I really know how I would feel? I was dealing with my fears, frustrations, and my ponderings over what it may be like. In the end, there was some control, but not a lot. Do you want 'em or not? A cup or DD's? Tattoos for nipples, or skip it? At least I had some time to decide everything. The whole process takes about a year. Lots of healing in that year. Lots of stretching in that year.

Stretching ... not only in body and mind, but also in Spirit. This takes trusting in God to a whole different level. Right now, I had to admit, I was a bit angry with God. Good thing he's big enough to handle that. I still love Him. I am just angry with some of the things He's allowed to happen in my life. Things I didn't understand, things that had been hurtful, things that had allowed pain—like the loss of my daughter and my marital difficulties.

Do I trust Him? On Monday, I would not have hesitated to say yes. As of yesterday, I had had to concede to "I'm trying to." It's not so much that I was trying to trust Him but that I was trying to trust that any more pain I had to endure would be for the right reasons. And what if I were trying to do the right thing and it all goes wrong? I'm trying to do what was His will for me. Some things had gone so wrong when I thought I was in His will. I mostly didn't trust myself to hear Him and know that if those things went wrong, it was not because of me. Or maybe it was supposed to go that way for me to learn a lesson. Maybe the lesson wasn't for me, but I was part of the lesson. The problem was, I would not know in this lifetime. I had to be OK with that. We all do.

The one good lesson cancer gives us is to re-evaluate our lives, our priorities, our choices. To not take for granted what we had was paramount. I learned that lesson when my vision suddenly began to fail last summer. I began to realize what an incredible gift it was to see the individual petals on a chrysanthemum and to enjoy what its color was. Discovering that it was a medication that caused the sight loss was a true miracle. I did have my sight return, most of it. I had lost a bit, but not much. In dim light, I had trouble telling the difference between blue and purple, orange and pink. Sometimes I need reading glasses, sometimes not. I couldn't see as well in the dark. But I was so grateful for the fact that I could see, that I didn't care that I had to adjust.

In the same manner, I knew I was so happy we found the cancer early that I could do this all hopefully without chemo or radiation, and be OK again. But, like the bit of vision I had lost, I would lose a bit of myself as well to the cancer.

I used to suffer from depression, and the big lesson I learned in that was how to be joyful in all circumstances. That was one of the hardest lessons to learn. It does not mean you were happy all the time. It means you do not allow yourself to block out the beauty and joy and good all around you in the midst of your grief.

Trust me, I've been there and the tendency was to say "WHAT good?" especially when someone you love was taken from you. Take a deep breath. Could you? Could you take a deep breath? Those suffering from lung cancer could not. Those suffering from congestive heart failure could not. Could you be thankful, grateful that you could take a deep breath? Feel how wonderful it really feels to take that deep, deep breath. Blow it out slowly and feel the tension release in your body, even if only for a moment.

Then look at the sky. The blue of the sky (or in my case this morning, the cloudy, gray, snowy sky), and be grateful that you could see it. Someone who could not see could not tell you if it was blue or gray in the sky today. They could not tell you if there were storm clouds or if they were the big beautiful puffy white cotton ball clouds. Maybe there was that glorious, frightening thunderhead in the distance. Could you watch it roll in? Be glad you could.

In Haiti there was a terrible earthquake. It caused so much sadness, so much devastating destruction, so much loss. The loss continues as they struggle to get aid to everyone. People were dying waiting for aid. Be grateful that you were not in the midst of it, and that we care enough about others to try to help, even if only in prayer. Could you be grateful for that too?

Do I grieve in all this? Of course. I would be a fool if I didn't. But my grief was not in the fact that I had cancer.

Take care, breathe deep, admire the color of the sky, and just do the next thing.

I grieve for the hold this disease would put on my life, delaying my plans, my dreams. I grieve for the loss of my God-given body parts. I grieve that I had to go through at least three surgeries that year, and that means IV's—my worst nemesis.

Too bad I'm only thick skinned in the epidermal sense.

Take care, breathe deep, admire the color of the sky, and just do the next thing.

Friends and Hope

Today, as I had been for the past week, I was in a bit of a fog. I just couldn't quite concentrate on things. Granted, I had reason to feel this way. It just amazes me how my upcoming surgery was affecting me. I'm totally oversleeping, not so much over eating (although I expect that). Lots of praying to understand; not so much why, but why now? Why, when I've already been through so much grief in the past few years did this have to hit now? How does this really have to change my life?

I had discovered, within the last year and a half, who my friends really were, and that was beyond measure, and makes this road quite a bit easier because I already knew who would be there when I needed someone. For someone who has lived the military lifestyle and moved twenty times in her life, having roots, real roots, was incredible. The wanderlust part of me that I had inside that helped me adjust, and survive, and enjoy all those moves was all but squelched by the knowledge that I didn't want to be away from these people I had grown close to and loved. It amazed me also how much more it hurt now when they moved away. It used to not bother me, and I could still be bad about keeping in touch, but it was so much harder when I had really gotten to know them. Now I understood all those new military wives, who had never moved before, and how scared they really felt when they moved. Now I understood.

One of my dear friends, and my mind was so fogged I could not remember which one (geez), was apologizing for telling me her troubles because they were so much less than mine. Remember, dear ones, that all our problems are big to us! Regardless of how big they are to others. I may have some days where someone's "lesser troubles" irritate me, but that was a personal problem. It was my problem. Just because I was going through stuff didn't mean the rest of the world was suddenly OK for everyone else. It was not OK to discount others' situations because yours may be "worse."

One of my dear friends had a disease that was terminal. Its progress was slow, and they expected her to have a normal life span, but it was terminal, there was   n   o cure, and no treatment other than trying to battle the symptoms. Her problems were bigger than mine in my estimation. We talked about our issues. She knew me better than anyone else at that point in time.

A diagnosis of cancer is not an automatic death sentence.

Talk to me, it's OK. I've only cried in front of two people (OK, maybe three), and they were actually not even over the cancer diagnosis. I had other issues, too. Other issues that bothered me more than the cancer did. The cancer affects those problems, but they didn't all just go away when the cancer decided to move in. And neither does anyone else's problems.

I'm trying to enjoy my coffee. It still tastes like coffee, and I was praying I would not have to take chemo when coffee no longer tastes like coffee. Even if I did, it would be temporary. Life goes on. One of my (other?) friends mentioned she was excited to meet the friend I was becoming when I got there. I wanted to meet her too. Where I would be in five years has been blown out the window. Or has it? I didn't know what dreams to still hold on to. Some of those dreams required a strength and a health that I may not have anymore. Maybe I was fretting for nothing. Maybe I would uncover a side of myself that really could conquer the world. The cancer could have my breasts, but it could not have my spirit. But that spirit was taking "a bit of a beating" for now. Maybe it was the waiting.

Waiting to know when surgery was. Waiting to go through surgery. Waiting to go through recovery. Waiting to know how I (my breasts) would feel. Waiting to know if we did get it all. Waiting to know when I could start really working on my own dreams. Waiting to know if it was time to get new dreams.

Waiting for this blasted foggy head to lift so I could at least do my assignment in my nutrition class. Part of me just didn't give a rat's butt about school anymore because I was so mad that I still couldn't proceed like I wanted to.

Waiting for the blasted fog to lift so I could get off my butt and clean my very neglected house. OK, well, maybe that fog could stay a bit longer, I didn't want to clean anyhow. Maybe some fairy would come and clean it for me. Hey, one could hope, right? Maybe some fairy could come and just beat her wand over my sons' heads and got them to at least pick up after themselves. Again, one could hope, right?

Hope. Never lose hope. Sometimes it is very elusive, but do not lose it. Hope may change, but do not give it up. Sometimes it's all we have. Right now, I had hope that I would be OK. I was just not sure anymore what "OK" was supposed to look like. I guess we'd find out when I got there.

Jell-O and Flying Prostheses

Raising teenage boys is like nailing Jell-O to a tree. Ain't it the truth? The pit that was my home seemed worse, dirtier, lately, but I had no idea if that was because (a) it was, (b) it just seems worse because I didn't have the energy to pick up after them, or (c) it's the same as always, I just notice it more right now. A plus about having one child, as opposed to two, was that they absolutely could not get away with blaming the dog for getting out the peanut butter and leaving it all over the counter, nor could they say it was the dog's turn to clean the bathroom or sweep the floor.

I think it's impossible (OK, "highly unlikely") to feel like a good parent when you are the one who is sick. When you are sick, you have to take care of yourself first. Which means: kids are no longer the primary concern to you. You are the primary concern for you. As a mom, that just didn't feel right. It didn't matter that both the boys were now teenagers, and relatively self-sufficient. I still had to cook, shop, care, and provide for them. It's tough to do when you need to be cared for:

Could it be that the cat was standing on my boob?

especially when you are in the single mom role, or in my case, the spouse of a deployed military man. It's tough. Not for the faint of heart.

I find that every new pain makes me jump a bit. What if the cancer is spreading? That pain was right where the cancer is, was that the cause of this pain? Was it still the pain from the biopsy site? Could it be that the cat was standing on my boob?

I had a funny revelation a few days ago. Because I would still keep the majority of the skin of my breasts (think hollowed out melons—guys, stop laughing, please), I would still have the scars from the sites of my biopsies (there were two), and the chickenpox scar (which looks just like a biopsy scar), as well as a few freckles and moles. Makes me think of that drink where you take a watermelon, hollow it out, take the insides and puree them with alcohol, and serve it in the watermelon. The outside was the same, but wholly cow, the inside was definitely not. Perhaps I should have one of those drinks. Maybe not.

I may be bummed about the school issue, but my cats were sure happy about it. I'm home more, which means more lap time. Boy were they going to be mad when I kicked them out after surgery. No lap time for about two weeks, so I was told. We shall see.

My son Alex asked me why I want to get reconstruction rather than just prostheses. The main reason was that I do not want to have to wake up in the morning and go "now where did my boobs go?" But I do have to admit, the idea of mortifying my boys with prosthetics would be hysterical. Picture it: They would be mouthing off to me in front of friends (eh, could happen) and I whip out a boob and wing it at them. I believe they would think twice about doing that again. I bet they would never bring anyone home ever again either.

Gee, would you consider that a plus or a minus here?

Oh, I had another reason I thought of for not getting prostheses. My dog. I have a Golden Retriever. He's the best dog: easy going, a bit lazy, and undemanding. Doesn't chew things up, he's totally housebroken, loves the cats. Like I said, he's a great dog. His only issue? In true Golden form, he constantly has to have something in his mouth. I never know what that might be. It's usually shoes, or a stuffed animal. He doesn't chew anything up, as I said, but he has to have something in his mouth. He even sleeps with something in his mouth. It's quite cute. Oddly enough, he usually barks with something in his mouth as well. He often carries around the dirty socks and underwear the boys do not put in the clothes hamper. I need to teach him how to put them in the laundry basket. Boy would that save me a lot of time!

That being said, remember, I lose stuff. I didn't want to wake up in the morning and not know where my boobs are. Even more, I do not want to wake up to the dog carrying them around the house. I'm not sure what the boys would think was worse, me winging a boob at them in front of their friends, or the dog bringing their friends my boobs. Neither was a pretty sight. Both would be traumatic not only for my boys, but for any poor recipient of such a "gift." My dog especially loves our Schwann's home food delivery man. That guy always gives my dog a treat. So, consequently, the dog brings him gifts too. Connect the dots, people. Poor Schwann's man.

I misplace things … a lot. Those who know me well know that I rarely go out of the house without having to go back in at least once because I forgot something: I misplace my keys, or phone, or purse, or shopping list, or wallet, or … you got the idea. So along those lines, I knew I would misplace my boobs if they were not attached. Same goes for my head. So I decided to not go the way of prostheses, although that would lessen the number of surgeries. Yes, I admit part of the rationale for me was cosmetic. I never thought I would be seeing a plastic surgeon. But it's a personal choice for every woman in my shoes.

Now I had grown up with them lying around the house, sometimes unattended. On that note, I had a funny idea to compile a list of funny things that I had heard, or seen, or thought of that were funny in the course of having prosthetics. Some were real, some were fictional. I would let you had the fun of figuring out which was which!

Top 25 Things to Do with Prosthetic Boobs

1. Had an impromptu game of fetch with the dog.
2. Throw it at your doctor when he delivers more bad news.

3. Pretend you own a voodoo parlor and walk around with straight pins sticking out of them while you wear them. (Especially effective in answering the door to a salesman)
4. They make great stress balls, for either you or hubby.
5. They make good floatation devices, especially in hot tubs.
6. When you had to have your son put on your dress so you could tailor the bottom, he could wear the boobs too so you got a more accurate hem line.
7. When you "had a headache," you could give them to him to play with so you could go to bed.
8. Piercings that didn't hurt.
9. You could now had removable/replaceable tattoos and even different ones if you had multiple sets of prosthetics.
10. Play catch at the park, even if you forgot the ball.
11. Use them to scare off little kids.
12. Use them to scare off unwanted men.
13. Use them to scare off teenagers.
14. Wear them on the outside of your shirt, and go to Mardi Gras.
15. Pacifiers
16. When it's cold, ear muffs.
17. When it's noisy, headphones.
18. Try on bras without actually trying on bras.
19. Throw them at your kids when they misbehave in public. (the threat of this alone usually works)
20. Scare off the daughter's new boyfriend.

21. Leave them laying in the front yard, and see who notices.
22. Take them up to the Wal-Mart® customer service counter and demand a different pair.
23. Put straws through the center, wear a blonde wig, and tell everyone you've been turned into a Fembot. (ala Austin Powers movie)
24. Put one in the refrigerator to use as a cold pack.
25. Use them as bookends at the local book store and see how long it takes for someone to notice.

I met a gal yesterday who was also a patient of breast cancer. Her road was a lot worse and a lot scarier than mine. I wanted to be supportive, but I was terrified I would say the wrong thing. Here she was with no hair, weak, going through chemo that was making her so sick. What was I supposed to say? I was not making light of my own situation, but she was still wondering if she would live. I had no doubt that I would be fine. But I did not know what to say to her. Do I say that the pink stripe in my hair was for her too? It was.

So many breast cancer survivors do not have to lose their hair to be survivors. Yet we only notice the ones that do. If all of us who had breast cancer put a pink strip in their hair, I wonder how different Wal-Mart might look. I think it would boggle the mind to realize how many women, when you see them, had dealt with this. Every woman in my family, my age and older on my mom's side (save one, or two) would have a pink stripe.

Maybe I should start something. I guess you could say I was thinking pink.

Rats Naturally Die from Cancer

January 26th was the day I learned I had cancer. Was it a day I would remember for the rest of my life? Not sure yet. I mean, I would remember when I got cancer, but not necessarily the date or time. I've already forgotten the time ... oh, wait, it was about 1:30 p.m. Now I remember. I was video chatting with my hubby, Lee, when I got the call. Anyhow, I would not say it was the worst day in my life. Not by a long shot.

Today, I find out the date of my surgery. I hope. I want to know when this crap would leave my body, hopefully, forever. I want to know how much time I had left to be "whole." Even when I was no longer whole, I would be here, and once again (after all the healing was done), healthy. For that I was grateful. But would I remember the date? I had had other surgeries. I remember the months in which I had them, approximately. My hip surgery was in late January, I believe. My ankle surgery was in late February. My wisdom teeth were removed over Christmas break, I think. All of them were just a blip on my radar. Would this surgery become no more than that eventually? Just another blip on my radar?

It's been snowing off and on for about three days now. Very little accumulation, but just enough to be pretty and make the roads bad. All the more reason to stay inside. Today I was really distracted. I wanted today to be over. I wanted to know. It was a busy day. I had things to do. So why couldn't I get up and move? It was as if I had this magnetic attraction between my backside and this chair, I could not seem to leave this spot and get moving, except to get more coffee. That magnetic pull was slightly more powerful.

If the proper paperwork was in, then today I needed to drop my other classes. I'm still so bummed about it. I had the online nutrition class. Even that was a struggle right now. It was more of a struggle because I had so much I needed to change in my diet, but being a comfort eater, I was not in the mood to change anything about my eating. I could feel my pants filling out a bit, I knew I needed to adopt better habits, but my world just got turned upside down. I didn't want to deal with this too. I feel like a bit of a naughty, overtired toddler who didn't feel like giving up the toy. Didn't want to. Toddler's rule of acquisition number one: If I think it's mine, then it's mine! I think that piece of cheesecake is mine, so it's mine. Actually, not just the piece, but the whole thing: so just hand it over and maybe I won't hurt anyone. Now go away.

I'm tired of hearing how this food or that food MAY help to reduce cancer risks. I tried to eat those foods. Couldn't really agree in any way that it actually has helped.

Besides, I didn't eat the required 6 pounds of broccoli, 2 pounds of salmon, and 8 pounds of blueberries, and 3 bottles of red wine (oh, wait, that was heart disease) every day for the last ten years. I guess that explains it. Come on. Even people who have awesome health habits, eat right, and exercise STILL get cancer. No, I had not had the best diet, nor had I been exercising like I should, but I was not convinced that had I done so I would be in a different place than I was right now.

My poor instructors had to deal with my 'tude. Good thing I didn't have to directly interact with them. That way I could grumble away without offending them. I try not to come off grumpy in my writings for the class, but sometimes it's tough. I just hope I do not have to write anything about how a good diet reduces cancer risks. I probably would, so I hope they won't take it personally when I say the research was stupid. There was no way to conclusively determine that diet has jack squat to do with cancer.

Remember, people, what do researchers study? Lab rats. Well, here's a thing to think about with lab rats. First, the rats have a very short life span, so anything they want to determine, the researchers feed them a lot of. Does broccoli decrease cancer? Well, let's feed this rat nothing but broccoli and find out! Two years later, the rat seems to die of natural causes. OK, fine, equate that to humans: you had to eat over 6 pounds of broccoli a day for ten years or something like that, and maybe you won't get cancer. In the lab setting, they have no choice but to organize it that way.

The second problem with the rat theories? I have news for you people. Guess what most rats normally die from? CANCER. So you know all those tests that say hot dogs cause cancer, or this causes cancer, or that causes cancer? If all rats normally die of cancer, how could they really tell? All the research really tells us is what may delay or expedite the cancers we were already prone to.

Forgive my grumpiness when you recommend I eat more of this and less of that. I already had cancer, it was not like I was going to prevent it now. So, zip it and pass me my cheesecake.

Patience and Bathing Cats

Waiting was a virtue that I had never quite mastered. I hate to wait. I've gotten a ton better. I don't mind waiting in line. I don't mind waiting for the gas tank to get full (of course, I do mind watching the price get higher as I pump). I don't mind waiting for people in the commissary when it's crowded (that's the military grocery store for those of you non-military types). I don't mind waiting for people in line dropping off their kids at school. I don't mind waiting at the doctor's office ... unless it was waiting in the doctor's office, and that particular doctor was my surgical oncologist (cancer doctor).

Suddenly, I was that impatient, impulsive person I thought I grew out of years ago. I knew I had cancer, I knew we had caught it early, but when you tell me I had to wait how many weeks until I could get this crap out of me, prepare to duck and cover. Of course I was nice in the office. All bark, very little bite, that's me (unless you were my husband—sorry, dear ... or occasionally the boys—sorry, guys). So I leave the office and the ranting begins.

How long was I supposed to wait? Until the dang stuff spread? Why couldn't they get it out now? You know, like 0630 (6:30 in the morning) *tomorrow*. Could we, could we, huh? The schedule was based off the plastic surgeon's schedule. Great. I had to wait in line behind some bimbo getting her DDs, a nose job, and a butt lift while I had cancer. Gee, that makes me feel important.

Patience was out the window. My attitude was shot. I was grumpy. I was frustrated. I just wanted to know *WHEN I WOULD HAVE SURGERY!* If it takes so long to make the appointment with the plastic surgeon, then why didn't the office make the appointment back three weeks ago when they knew I would need an appointment? Why hadn't they made the appointment last week after I had already spoken to the plastic surgeon? What purpose did my appointment serve yesterday when nothing was accomplished that could not have been accomplished in a five-minute phone conversation? Nothing in that meeting that transpired would had made squat worth of difference in the date of my (YES, I WANT THIS) surgery. Why did anyone even ask that question to a cancer patient?

It also postpones the Red Cross and getting Lee home from Iraq so he could hold down the fort at home. Do they not realize how unbelievably taxing it was to worry that your husband was in a war zone there, while you were in a personal war zone with your own body here? Probably not.

I had a run-in with a nurse that severely impacted my relationship with my cancer doctor. This nurse had worked for him for a very long time. Crossing her would be like crossing my doctor, and even writing this story feels like I was crossing that line. However, I was in my right, so I shall share.

The Red Cross was working to get Lee home from Iraq, and one of the things they had to do was verify the diagnosis with one of my doctors. It made sense. That way you didn't get lonely spouses crying wolf all the time, just to have their husbands back home. That being said, there was a lot of "hurry up, and wait." Lots of things to be done, and quickly, because the chains of communication would be slow, and there were many people involved in the process of relieving him of duty, replacing him, arranging transportation home, etc. It was not something that happened over night.

The Red Cross had let me know they were having trouble getting in touch with my oncologist to verify my diagnosis, and asked if I could help. So I called the office, asked to be transferred to the nurse, and got voice mail. I called back and explained that I needed to talk to the nurse, not her answering machine, and could they please track her down. Yes, I would wait. She was not happy that I had interrupted her rounds and had no sympathy for trying to get my husband home. She told me she would talk to them after 1800 (6:00 p.m.). I informed her that would be too late. She said that she would not be available today to speak to the Red Cross. I couldn't believe it. Here I had just been diagnosed with cancer, and she, a cancer nurse, had no sympathy for the fact that my husband was sitting in a war zone, and we didn't even know if we could get him home. She was obviously not willing to assist me.

I persisted and asked if anyone else could talk to the Red Cross for her, and she snapped at me that she didn't even have the official report in her hands, so that I would just have to be patient. I was livid.

However, she had given me an idea. I knew beyond a shadow of a doubt who did have that report: my radiologist! I love my radiologist. I find her and her nurses to be wonderfully caring and patient, and considerate in times where every woman who comes through the door was stressed, unsure, and sometimes downright scared.

I called her office. I explained what happened to her secretary, who immediately paged my radiologist, who, in turn, got on the phone immediately and spoke to the Red Cross. Talk about angels on earth!

That instance was the second one I had had with Nurse Ratchet (as I came to call her).

I contacted the office manager and complained. I told her everything that had transpired between the biopsy, and the Red Cross, and informed her that I would appreciate it if I didn't have to deal with Nurse Ratchet again. I would like to say that was the end of it, and I did not have to see her again, but I did. However, it was obvious that she got the message, and she did tread more carefully around me after that. Truth be told, I would not have been the first person to change doctors because of poor nursing care. Had he not been the best doctor in the area, I would have. I made the decision to deal with Ratchet in lieu of knowing I was seeing the best doctor. I still think he should rethink his staffing choices.

So I waited.   And I tried to remind myself to have faith in the fact that God was ultimately in charge, and everything would work out as it was supposed to. This took faith, and trust in God to a totally different level for me. Obviously we had things we had to do in this life, choices we had to make. You know, like whether or not to throw our fake boobs at the human boobs in our lives.

However, how do you fathom the difference between what was your job and what was God's job?   Should I have the chocolate cake or the strawberry cheesecake? God's job or my job? (OK, I should pass on them both and have an apple. Fine.) Survive this time in my life: God's job or my job? I had a say in each, but that didn't mean I should always speak up. Sometimes all I succeed in doing is getting in His way and mucking it up.

It's kind of like giving a cat a bath. One experienced person was the wise choice to do this job. Adding an inexperienced person to the job would likely end with someone getting hurt (usually the experienced one). Yet, you let the inexperienced person help because how else were they supposed to get experience? But when that inexperienced person comes into it with an attitude of "I know better than you," it's always bad. How often do we do that to God? No, thanks, God, I got this one. I know myself, I know my limitations: I am in control here. You could just sit this one out.

Then God laughs. You know He did! Why wouldn't He laugh at us? We are that inexperienced moron who thinks he's smart enough to give a reluctant, fully-clawed cat a bath. Right. Go for it. That was about the time I would have sat back and enjoyed. I would let him struggle with the poor cat. Not worried about the cat. The cat was just fine taking care of himself, although he looks as frantic as I felt in dealing with the surgeons.

The guy wrestles and tries. The cat flails and scratches, and yowls to high heaven. The guy starts cussing and splashing, the cat starts tearing flesh, all the while the guy was saying his mantra, "I got this, I got this." You get the idea. And I sit back, smiling, and wait until he finally concedes he doesn't "got this." Inevitably he is soaking wet. That cat is probably pretty dry, and certainly not bathed. He's bleeding profusely, hair all messed up, bathroom all wet, and the cat, now looking quite smug, as he licks a paw in retort.

Then I step in, deftly grab the cat, and lickety split, before the cat even realizes it, he is bathed and under the dryer. I make it look easy. Of course, I have experience. I know how to do this. The guy, of course, was not happy as I then helped him bandage his wounds. He just couldn't understand why he was unsuccessful. It looked so easy. I made it look so easy. He thinks he's stronger than I and thinks he's wiser. Yet he failed. He neglected to realize that I knew what I was doing. Did he ask for my help? No. Did he acknowledge early on that he was in over his head? No. Did he turn the job over to me to handle? No. He did not concede until he was ripped up and totally humiliated by a seven-pound ball of fluff.

This time, I was that guy. I needed to shut up, quit trying to do it myself, ask for help, and acknowledge that God knows better than I. Someday I will learn that lesson. I sure hope I learn it fast.

Port

Getting a "by the way" from your doctor's nurse was not always a good thing. I did finally receive a surgery date yesterday. Hurrah! That really helped my mood and attitude. Like I said, I was not a patient person in this matter. Anyhow, I was feeling really good about finally having a date, but the stress did take its toll and I needed some rest. So I took a snooze.   I awoke to a message on my phone to the sound of Nurse Ratchet's voice saying,   "… and they would put in your port during surgery."

Port? Why would I need a port? So I call back, and they say I need a port for my chemo. Chemo? What chemo?

"Well, haven't you talked to Dr. So and so, and Dr. So and so?"

Nooooo. Didn't know I needed to talk to Dr. So and so.

"Oh, well didn't the doctor talk to you about this in your appointment on Tuesday?"

No, no he didn't.

"Oh…."

Oh. OK….well shoot. On the flip side, the silver lining, I would have a port. For those who were unaware of what a port was, it was a type of catheter they put in a large vein close to your heart rather than in a vein in your arm. It stays there for a longer time as opposed to a regular IV that has to be changed every forty-eight hours. It seems nasty, but the flip side was that you only had to have it done once (ideally). That means, I would not have to have fifty million IV attempts for however many times I had to go have chemo. That was a good thing, people! I had very uncooperative veins. They didn't like IV's. They roll, hide, blow, and, to top it off, I had an elephant's hide tough skin. I liked the idea of a port.   So I was happy about that. I had always expected chemo as much as I always expected cancer. I did, however, fear the IV's and chemo. Now that the IV was not an issue, I was good.

Of course, I still had an IV for surgery. Rats. Oh well. The other plus to the port was that the chemo would not be frying my veins in my hand and arm. That was also a good thing. Remember the blown vein during my MRI? That was over a month ago. Today was the first day my hand and arm no longer hurt. I couldn't imagine how badly a chemo infiltration would burn. I'll take the port.

As I laugh with friends about all the wonderful fun I could have had with prosthetic boobs, I was almost sorry I'm not going that route. Perhaps vanity was winning out over humor. Or perhaps I want to wear a normal bra and a normal bathing suit. But I had to admit that just the deterrent of flying boobs might really make the boys shape up, especially if I got piercings per the recommendation of a friend. I'm not into body piercings, but piercing fake boobs wouldn't bother me. So picture flying boobs with piercings in them. Intriguing.

I've been looking at the possible meds I would be put on. As usual, don't let the long lists of possible complications scare you. Just read the box of aspirin. So I expect to feel like crap, maybe have sinus infections, and perhaps lose my hair. Nothing unexpected. There were scarier things, but the chances of those were low, so, I'm not worried. Not sure how long I would have to do this, but it sure may complicate things for "my plans."

Wow. That thought, "my plans," makes me really start to laugh. They were not plans anymore, merely suggestions, desires. What plans I had were going to be given to me. Good thing I was not a total control freak. In a way it was nice to just be told "this was what you would do." Too bad what I had to do was going to be uncomfortable. But it was only for a time, and I would reach the other side. I was just hoping for simple.

What plans I had were going to be given to me.

In giving myself a break from it all, I was going to go to the zoo. I love the zoo, the sounds and even the smells. Nice break to forget the cancer, and all that was ahead of me, if only for a few hours.

Roller Coasters

In general, I am not a fan of roller coaster rides. I do not like feeling thrown around, or dropped, or going upside down. I'm a wimp. Hard to believe I wanted to be a pilot for years and never liked roller coasters. I guess it's a good thing I never did become a pilot. I get the feeling of turbulence when flying and I want to scream in stark terror and grab onto anything that is firmly nailed down, which on a plane during turbulence, nothing feels nailed down.

Besides, how many times have you gone to sit in a roller coaster ride, (you know, the really good ones) only to discover someone barfed in the seat? Yuck! No thanks. Or having to worry that someone behind you, or in front of you, would barf on you during the ride? What about those lovely cameras they have now to showcase and record people like me who are terrified of roller coasters? People on video shows are capitalizing on people like me with those shots. No thanks. Don't like roller coasters, don't like flying. I like my feet firmly on the ground, thank you very much!

Yet, somehow, emotional roller coasters are different. Thank goodness! This is probably due to not screaming like a little girl on the way down, even though I do feel my heart drop just as much. Then again, the going up, the thrill, the anticipation, the pure joy, yeah, it's there!

What a day yesterday. Yesterday, I woke up knowing I was going to have chemo, not knowing if/when/how long Lee was going to be home.   Yesterday morning I was frustrated, tired, and grumpy. Today I got to wake up knowing I was not having chemo, Lee was being sent home, and would not have to go back to Iraq, and there was a good possibility he may be home by next weekend.

I truly was happy that Lee was coming home. It was a bizarre roller coaster of emotions all on its own. I was happy I would not be doing this alone, but I was still so mad, I didn't want him in the house, yet. It was going to be nice to have him there to help out with the boys, the cooking, shopping, etc.

There was a wonderful peace with knowing the answers, knowing the time frame. Joy, peace.

Yes, there were days that I was frustrated, but that was OK. I would be worried if those days didn't happen. Either way, I was grateful for the stability in my life: my friends, family, the cats, my dog, the fact that the sun rises, even if only above the clouds.

I could hardly wait for spring and the leaves to return to the trees and to take long walks outside, rather than on the treadmill or on a track indoors. Going through this all was really kind of like winter. It's cold, yucky, uncomfortable, and some days you really don't want to get out of bed, but you know that if you just hang on, spring would come. Hopefully, sans the Midwest tornadoes.

This was part of where faith comes in, I believe. Or maybe I should say the "joy in all circumstances." I knew that it would all work out in the end. I had that faith. I was not ignorant of the pit falls, but I chose to try not to worry about them since it would not change their reality. Besides, I was missing the joy of today when I gave in to the sorrows and fears and pain. I was not successful with this every day, but I was more successful than not.

I look at myself in the mirror and know I will be OK. Life was good. It was changing, even minute by minute, but it was good. That was good enough for today.

Battlefields

How do you prepare your spouse for something like this? I mean, yes, I would live, but it changes the dynamics of the physical relationship a bit. I had tried to always prepare Lee for this eventuality, and he thought he was. When we were still early in our relationship I used to say, "Enjoy them now, they won't be here forever!" I think he was going to be surprised that this would be harder than he thinks. It's sure turning out to be harder for me than I thought, and it's my body this was happening to. I had heard of relationships where this had huge, negative implications on the marriage. Breasts were important to guys. No, it may not be the most important thing, but for some guys, they could not handle the scars, the "deformity" (let's be real people, they would never look right after this). In clothes, I look normal. Out of clothes, I would be different. That was life. Many men actually leave their wives because they could not handle it. How sad is that? I feel proud to be around men who think otherwise and don't let the scars of the body scar the relationship.

In a way, I like scars. They were as much a sign that I had lived as battle scars were for soldiers. They mean something. I fought. I survived. I lived.   That was something to be proud of. But, unlike a soldier's battle scars, there was no cool story to go with it. It's not like I could regale an audience with a "There I was …" kind of heart stopper. Then again, perhaps I could do what my brother did. Sorry, Ed, I have to tell this story. I love this story.

When my brother was in college, he went in for surgery on the varicose veins on his legs. They removed some moles as well and found skin cancer. It was caught just in the nick of time, but they had to do some pretty radical surgery on his knee where the mole was, as well as remove the lymph nodes in his more private areas. So he's got some fun scars as well. Anyhow, due to the varicose vein surgery and the cancer surgery, he has a ton of scars up and down his legs with a wicked one on his knee.

As I said, he was in college. He was at University of California, Santa Barbara, and he volunteered at the marine biology lab, where they took kids on tours. He was taking some kids around and there was an area with small sharks, about a foot long. They were small enough to handle to show the kids, so he had picked one up. It managed to scratch him on the finger with a tooth, causing a small cut. It healed fine, but left a little scar. So, when he was on the beach, and someone asks where he got all the scars, he tells him he was bitten by a shark. I love it.

He's got a cool story. Granted, my mom didn't have a cool story, and she has more scars than I would. However, the number of times she has beaten cancer is pretty impressive. How many, you ask? No idea. I lost track. At least three battles with breast cancer, and who knows how many from skin cancer, thyroid cancer, etc. It's like a perpetual boxing match for her. She's won every round, but doggone it, couldn't seem to KO the stupid thing. But she's still alive and kicking. By now, I would say she has a story to tell.

Lee has to go from duty in Iraq to duty at home with a sick wife. Lucky him. No time for transitioning. No time for changing gears, no time for readjusting. No time for retraining for his new duties. He's going to have quite a time. He was not going to be available to go anywhere for a while. Although that was fine for us, it's part of his job to go places. This would change that.   He's been in the Air Force over seventeen years. Was he going to be done deploying? Was he going to have to give up the part of the job he loves most? That was a lot to ask of a man. That, on top of knowing he's got a sick wife who was also going to be going through menopause and the total roller coaster associated with that, as well. He's exchanging one battlefield for another. Time would tell which one proved to be more volatile. I feared it would be the one ahead.

In other words, he was trading one combat zone for another one. I was very aware as I wrote this that I was feeling very torn knowing he was willing to take this on with me, even though I had asked for a divorce. I was relieved he chose to stay and tackle this with me, come what may. Yet I was still so mad at him, part of me didn't want him anywhere near me. How do you balance that? But I was still so set on my course that I refused to admit to myself that I was really worried about how the surgery would change things. Secretly, I was worried that he wouldn't find me attractive anymore, and if he didn't, no man would, I feared. Of course, why should I care if I wanted a divorce? Hmm, could you smell that conflict going on inside me? I couldn't. I was being blind. I was spending so much energy being mad that I was denying the obvious fact that I still cared. Yup, I was totally lost and confused.

Prime Rib and Running Shoes

I'm one of those emotional eaters. I remember buying my off-the-shoulder wedding dress too big because I expected to gain at least ten pounds between the time I bought it and the time of the last alteration. It was a size 6. In that particular instance, I was quite wrong. I did drop about five pounds by the time of the last alteration. No biggie, but it was taken in as far as it could be without destroying the lace and beading on the dress. That was one week before the wedding. By the wedding, I had dropped another ten pounds, and my off-the-shoulder dress fell frighteningly to the ground when I exhaled. I remember putting on a long-line bra and quickly sewing in about three bra pads (or so it seemed) in each side. I had to maintain exquisite posture if I expected to stay clothed. And not exhale.

It was worse with my going-away dress. That dress was bought at a size 10, but I was not even in a size 4 at that point. It really fell right off me. One of my dear bridesmaids was unable to attend (Germany was a bit too far to come from for her at that time), and her dress was a size 6. It was also off the shoulder (what WAS I thinking?). So I had to, yet again, have perfect posture. The most comical photo of my wedding was when one of the groomsmen dumped a baggie of bird seed over my head (thanks, Gary!). Where did it go? Right down the front of my dress. The picture caught me as I was feeling all this birdseed go rolling into my bra. It's a cute picture. My husband had fun on our wedding night picking birdseed out of my hair and bra.

Like I said before, I am an emotional eater. This time, however, I doubt I would be losing any of that weight in a blessed turn of events. This time, I'm expecting to pack on a few. When you feel as stressed as anyone with cancer would, you find whatever comforts you. It makes me wonder how many smokers' and drinkers' addictions go nuts during these times. I was glad I did not have those to worry about.   But I eat and snuggle with my cats. I used to eat a ton back when I was running six miles a day. I kept eating that much after I had stopped (thanks to a surgery or two), and I have packed on more than a few. I'm not bad, mind you. I'm just slightly overweight. But I fear that my cravings for 16 ounces of prime rib, and brownies, and French fries all the time may be a problem. Top it off with my nutrition class. I think learning to eat healthy was making it worse. Now I look at stuff and go, "Holy cow! That thing of soup was half my day's salt!" Then I eat it anyhow, all day worrying about my salt intake. Or "Look at how much fat was in that!" And I eat it anyway and spend the day looking at my gradually spreading midsection. Then I do the same at dinner.

I walk, or at least I try to. I always seem to find 50 million other things I should be doing, as if walking was an incredibly expensive guilty pleasure I need to talk myself out of. "Oh, I'd love to spend an hour walking, but I really had to get the kitchen cleaned so I could cook dinner." Or the popular, "I didn't have time to walk, get all stinky, take a shower, and then be ready when the boys got home and have all their stuff we need to do."

I need to make time to exercise a priority. It needs to be sacred. It needs to be my own. How come I could carve out four hours to take classes each day, but when I had to drop them, I had no time for exercising? Didn't I understand what this was doing to my health? Didn't I have a clue how important this was? Well, yeah, I do have that clue. I'm not sure why it's so hard to get myself to walk. I had no excuse. I had a treadmill in the house. I even brought it upstairs so I would use it more often. It's even in front of the TV!

Now I would have to be concerned that I keep proper weight proportions with my new boobs. They would no longer lose weight when I do (and that was a good thing), nor would they get bigger if I gain. Add to that the ever-present reality of it being more difficult to lose weight after thirty-five (I'm there), and it's worse after menopause (I'll be there soon enough). So what was a girl to do, I asked myself.

Duh. Put down the fork and pick up the shoes and make some friends that I see only at the gym. Maybe that would motivate me. Because, heaven forbid, I should just do this for myself. Do I think I'm special or something? Yeah, I was. I'm worth it. And I would, admittedly, like to work myself into a smoking hot body to "prance around" and proclaim, "Surviving could look THIS good!"

One could hope. Or one could work. Now, where did I put my shoes? Hmm. There they were under that huge pile of laundry I've been meaning to get done.

Wresting Moves and Button-Down Shirts

Leave it to my boys to make me laugh. Not just a chuckle, but a good enough laugh to have me remembering it for days, and laughing all over again. Fred tries to make jokes, which often fall flat, but the attempts were hysterical in and of themselves. Alex, on the other hand, didn't try to be funny, but says such off-the-wall stuff, he was funny.

We were in the car, and I had just picked Alex up from wrestling practice. He was describing the techniques and take downs and all the little stuff that the uneducated would not see during a match. Did you know that they dig their chins into their opponents? It hurts. It's distracting, and a good hard throw down would cause your opponent to get just disoriented enough for them to say "screw it" for about the five seconds it takes to pin them.

Then, there was pinching, including the infamous "titty twisters." He had that one happen to him that day, and he was talking about how much it hurt. And I started laughing. Not because it hurt him, but because I realized that if I ever were to engage in a titty twister battle (not that I would), I would always win. Why? Because they would be fake! No nerves! Twist away, baby! The worst that could happen was that you twist them off. Not even sure that's possible, but what a hilarious thought! Gee, a sport I could excel at. Not one I want to participate in, but one I could excel at. Too funny!

My surgery was less than a week away. I was doing my final shopping, arranging the house, getting ready, and shopping for button-down shirts, sweatshirts and comfortable pull-on pants. I probably would not be able to dress myself at all for about a week. Lovely. That also meant help going potty. Fun. I simply would not have the upper body strength to pull my pants up and down. Nice. Oh well. I'd deal, and it would only be for a while.

The drains I would have were messy, unsightly, and probably going to ruin some clothes, so I was told. I would not be able to raise my hands or arms above my head for a while, and I was learning that pulling on shirts would be uncomfortable for a while—thus, the shopping trip. Power shopping was not my thing, but that was exactly what I did. A friend of mine and I went to the local Goodwill store and went nuts. I had an overflowing cart full of blouses, camisoles, sports tops, button-down shirts, button-down sweaters, and sweatpants. I was terrified what the bill was going to be. I was sure I would be spending like four hundred dollars or something, and I was cringing with each item the cashier rung up. The grand total? One hundred thirty dollars. Wow. What a relief. It was weird to buy an almost entirely new wardrobe in one shot.

See, I hate button-down shirts. I always feel like they gap in the wrong places, so I really didn't have many, and the ones I did have I was not willing to get stained, or they would be too small with the swelling that was going to be happening. I had bought an entire closet full of clothes just for this … I felt guilty, because I do not need this many clothes. But then I reminded myself that I do, but only for now. I would see what clothes survived this and then pass them along. Maybe another cancer patient could use them. I liked that thought.

I just got the final notification: Lee gets home from Iraq today. That was a huge weight off my mind. I needed to be able to concentrate on the surgery ahead, not have to worry each day whether or not he's safe. It was time to go get the finishing touches and final shopping done before he arrived. Always short notice. Welcome to the military!

Did you hear that? I was happy not to have to worry about whether he was safe. Does that really sound like a woman ready for a divorce, does it? I mean, I picture women who were really ready for divorces to pretty much wish their husbands would just drop over dead, and they meant it. Although I had moments where I thought that, I immediately felt guilty because I knew he was a good person, even if I felt he hadn't been a good husband. Of course, I also had not had the biggest "duh" realization until about a year later, which was simply that just like you could be a great parent, and have a bad parenting moment (we all have), by the same token, you could have bad spousal moments, but still be a great spouse. No one was perfect, but I was so convinced that Lee was capable of being perfect, and that he just didn't feel like working that hard. Instead, I needed to give him credit for being human, imperfect, fallible, and allow him permission to make mistakes. Mistakes that sometimes hurt deeply, but were never intentional.

My confusion was at an all-time high. I was so mad, I didn't want to look at him. I didn't want him to touch me, but at the same time, I knew I had just a few days until surgery, and a certain part of my sexuality would be forever gone. I wanted to be touched one last time. I felt conflicted, and selfish, because I wanted to be touched, but not by Lee. I didn't want to be touched by anyone else, but I didn't want him to touch me either. So I felt like asking to be touched was very selfish. At the same time, I had two things running through my head: If I didn't, I would never feel this ever again, and secondly, how could I do that emotionally to Lee? I had asked him for a divorce, I wasn't wearing my ring, I had kicked him out of the bedroom, but I had the nerve to ask him to touch me? I tried to rationalize to myself that he wouldn't care, he was a guy, and an invitation to cop a feel was just that, an invitation, and he wasn't likely to pass it up. Although I may have been correct, I didn't want him to think that I was in any way changing my mind. I was so confused, frustrated, and scared, and I wouldn't even admit it to myself.

The Big Day

Well, you could knock me over with a feather! I woke up this morning after another so-so night's sleep. Fed the cats, fed the dog, fed the birds, and struggled to NOT make myself a "cuppa jo." Today was surgery day. I was going to sit down and write one more note, pre-surgery, but thought I would check Facebook first.

I was overwhelmed! Three of my dear friends from high school, Keelie, Kay, and Julie, had taken it upon themselves to put pink in their hair! One of my friends even put pink in her daughters' hair: all in support. I love them so much! That was wonderful that they chose to support me in this way. See, all of us were, well, not known for this kind of expression. I think only Kay would had said "cool!" when we were in high school. (It makes me chuckle at the memories.) It was overwhelming. This has been a trying time, and the support I had received meant so much. I had never felt as many prayers, as much love, or as much support as I had while going through this. I could not explain how much it meant!

I was really not very nervous or anxious for anything about today except that I was dying for my coffee. I was such a creature of habit here. I had my routine. I was not looking forward to getting the IV catheter put in, but that was the only thing. I was packed. I had magazines to occupy my time before my surgery. I had a nice big, fluffy, warm blanket so I did not freeze at the hospital, as I'm always cold in hospitals. I went in with the knowledge that I was totally surrounded by the prayers of my friends and family. What was there to worry about? This morning, I had cancer. Tonight, I would be cancer free. This was a good thing.

This morning, I had cancer. Tonight, I would be cancer free.

And here was where I usually pause, take a big sip of coffee, warm my hands, and contemplate the next minute or so. OK, I need to pack some of my coffee. That was one of the first things I would want after surgery (if I'm not throwing up or anything).

When we lived in Seoul, South Korea, I was introduced to these coffee "sticks." Something similar has just recently come out here. It was basically individual servings of instant coffee in little prepackaged sticks. I love them. You could buy them at the Asian food stores. So my morning routine includes one to two cups of coffee made with these little sticks of coffee. My mouth was just watering for a cup right now. I feel like Homer Simpson when he sees a doughnut and starts slobbering and saying "glazed" or whatever it was he says. Sorry, guys, not a Simpsons fan, but you get the idea.

I tried to tank on the water last night, for the sake of my veins and eat a good meal so that I wouldn't have my tummy growling like crazy. Although I was not too happy about waiting so long for my surgery (it's at one thirty), I was really happy it wasn't early this morning, because I would have worried all night about over sleeping (which I never do anyhow, so why I was worried was beyond me). I slept as well as I could, with little worry or anxiety about the surgery today. Didn't sleep well anyhow, but that was about normal. Maybe I'm just getting "older" and didn't need as much sleep anymore. Maybe my body was betraying my anxieties that I do not seem to be thinking, or feeling, but was still affecting my sleep. Eh, whatever. It's all good.

In the face of all the malpractice, etc., they now mark on you which side the surgery side was, and which side the surgery was not. I thought I would have a bit of naughty fun and mark on various body parts that they were either not to be touched, or (in the case of my derriere) they could feel free to take a bit if they so choose. I plan to put "not yet" over my ovaries as that was the next surgery. I didn't go totally over-board, but I think it should lighten up things a bit. I'll see you soon with a little bit less of myself.

Post-Surgery Day 3

I'll write a quick note while the room isn't spinning quite so fast (I love pain meds). The surgery could not have gone smoother. Everything was textbook. The nurses were all fabulous. They got my IV in on the first shot (HURRAH!), and there were no complications. About the only thing was that I took forever in recovery. I was in surgery for about four hours, and recovery for about four hours … I guess I was tired.

I was able to get up almost immediately. I had some numbness in the hand on the right side where they did the lymph node biopsy. I guess they bumped a nerve. It happens. That should improve soon. Good thing I am left handed! I had pretty limited movement of my arms for a while. I felt like I tried to (unsuccessfully) bench press two hundred pounds. I was sore, but not in any real pain.

The drains were ugly, a bit cumbersome, but they really did not bother me. It's actually fascinating watching the drainage turn from the red, to orange to now getting close to yellow. These were good things. It means great healing was taking place.

My head was pretty fuzzy from the meds, but that too would go away. I'm being very well taken care of. Well, "taken care of" consisted of Lee taking good care of me, and even so, I wasn't about to give him that credit. He was doing a great job, especially in such a hostile environment, but I wasn't about to let him know it. Nor was I going to let myself know it, either.

The cats were being pretty respectful, and not trying to get up on my chest at all. I was not up to going to church today only because I knew I'd fall asleep during the service, and I didn't want to be rude.

Oh, and most exciting, I WAS CANCER FREE!

Red to Yellow

I'm gradually getting off the pain meds. Hurray! That means not only was I getting better, it also meant the head was clearing as well, and I was not spending all day sleeping, or trying to stay awake. I look a bit like a borg, ala Star Trek, with the tubes coming out of me. Sorry, not tubes, but drains.

The TV series *Star Trek, Next Generation* had a villainous species that were half human, half machine. They thought with one mind, called the collective. The quote they always used was, "Resistance is futile. You will be assimilated." Their bodies were made up of partial machine parts, most notably tubes in replace of veins. These tubes were on the outside of the body. I suppose they were insinuating that when you were assimilated you no longer needed blood, but oil or something. I have no idea, but they were ugly, and right about then, I felt as if I had been assimilated.

The drains were a bit irritating only because they pull, and that hurts. They were now "healed" to my body, so removing them would be interesting. I was not sure if I needed to be putting anything on them to keep the skin looser, but I could ask the doctor at my appointment tomorrow.

It was interesting watching the fluid draining out of me. It's not that it was gushing or anything, or that I could actively watch it, but the color changed as I was healing. It went from a red (mostly blood) to an orange, which was a combo of plasma and blood, to yellow which was plasma. Now, I was still at the orange stage, but I could see it getting lighter each day, which was wonderfully encouraging.

Since it was uncomfortable to even hold a book right now, I was catching up on all sorts of TV I didn't know (or care) that I was missing. I found that I really enjoyed *Monk*, and *Psych* (Fred loves that show, now I finally started watching it). But I am not watching quite as much *NCIS* as I expected. Probably because it isn't on as much as the others. Whatever. I'd rather be reading or writing, or talking to everyone. I got a lot of phone calls as well.

The weather was finally getting nice. Translation: it was above freezing, and the sun could be seen. The birds were out more, and I could hear them singing when I poked my head out the door as Buddy, our dog, goes out to do his business. Perhaps I could take a walk today. I'd probably make it about two houses and turn around and come back, but that would be two houses farther than yesterday. Go, me!

I was excited to hear from the doctor what things I could start trying to do as I started to feel better. I wondered what types of stretching I would be starting with, and when I would get my stitches out. Or, better yet, when would I be getting my tubes out. I think that was dependent on the amount of fluids they kick out in a given day (we measure that two times a day).

Well, my window of alertness was drawing to a close for the moment, so I would sign off. I would drift off into dreamland until something else awakens me, and I get to try to stay awake once more.

Peristalsis

Whew, it's been a few days! Although my last entry was definitely more awake, and coherent, I was definitely not prepared to go off the pain meds that early. I paid for it. Boy, did I. Lesson learned. I would deal with the fogginess. After all, it was only a week since I had had major surgery. Getting a bit over ambitious, wasn't I? Not out of character for me at all. OK, you can stop laughing now.

The color changes in my drains were still gradually going from red to yellow, definitely more yellow than red today, and the volume was saying I was getting closer! I do feel in general better. The only issue, which was a concern, was that the peristalsis (that's what you call the movement of the intestines) was practically at a standstill. Translation: constipation. It's not a matter of "quality" here, but motility, movement. It turns out that my intestines were rather sleepy too. I'm not really uncomfortable (yet), but the lack of production would warrant a trip to the Doctor's office where he would ask me if I had been drinking lots of water. Yes. Eating prunes? Yes. Moving around? Yes, as much as I was comfortable moving. Taking the stool softeners? Yes. Eating roughage? Yup. Had I tried an enema? Yes, more than one.

I had to make sure I gave Lee major kudos here in regard to the enemas. Guess what? I could not administer them alone. Poor Lee had to truly "put it where the sun didn't shine" for me. How disgusting was that when you had a good relationship with the person? We may say "put it where the sun doesn't shine!" in anger, but I guarantee that was not the intention. However, bless his heart, he wrinkled up his nose, did his best not to throw up, and helped me with these little procedures, more than once. And yet, I still wasn't giving him credit for doing a good job caring for me.

Yup, I know, I'm an idiot.

I was not sure what was next to relieve the pressure. The pharmacist, who was informed about all the meds I'm on, suggested a light laxative. OK, whatever. Better than a trip back to the hospital which seemed to promise some rather uncomfortable procedures, top of the list was another IV.

Lovely.

I had all these meds to help ease my pain, and keep me healthy, but all meds had side effects. I was on pills to help those side effects, which in turn had side effects of their own. Meanwhile, other members of my family were catching whatever the current creeping crud was. My son Alex came down sick today. He's got a fever, headache, and body aches.

Well, the meds were kicking in again, so I was going to sign off. Hopefully all this would pass (all pun intended).

Tubes

They removed the tubes, and I no longer look like Borg. Now, I want to describe the experience in a bit of detail that may not be for the squeamish. So if graphic detail is not your cup of tea, you may want to pass on reading this. The purpose of this TMI (too much information) kind of note was because I hope to have as much detail of my experience to pass on to other survivors, and new cancer patients to give a better idea of what REALLY happens, at least in my case. That being said, here we go.

The thing about the drains, for me, was that they were terribly uncomfortable. A lot of the reasons for the pain meds had to do with the drains. They are sewn into your body, but their natural inclination (due to weight of fluid in them and gravity) was to pull out. So, you had this tug of war going on between the sutures trying to keep the drains in, and gravity and your body trying to pull them out. After about 10 days, they were so uncomfortable that any way I moved seemed to irritate them. It was annoying. It's not a searing, "holy cow I hurt" kind of pain, but more like someone constantly pulling on one hair on your forearm, and it hurts. You remember those fights with your siblings when you were little and they would pull the hair on your arms? Oh, how it hurt! Then you would usually resort to hitting them just to keep them from pulling your hair.

Come to think of it, the hair pulling was how I used to "defend" myself from my brothers when I was little, when they would pin me to the floor and tickle me. They would gang up on me (remember this, guys?) and I was told by my dad (thanks dad) to pull the hair on their legs. Oh boy, did that work. I didn't get ganged up on much after that.

The drains oozed around the sides. It was not blood, but plasma, the kind of clearish, yellow stuff. It was slimy at first, got all over everything, and then when it dried was crusty and pokey. The oozing was not profuse, but pretty constant (for me). I got it on my clothes, so I would wear a part of a maxi pad underneath it to absorb the leakage, and I would tape that in place with medical tape I had at home. It was bulky, but it kept me dry and feeling less goopey.

That was what my drains felt like. So I got into my cancer surgeon's office for my check up with him, and he takes a quick look at me and the sutures on my breasts, we go over the time line for future surgeries (the ovary removal), and when we would start the cancer preventative drugs (OK, this set of drugs and when to take them was a note for another time: "Why give them AFTER cancer when a patient has the cancer gene?"). I asked if he could remove the drains. He told me that the plastic surgeon does that.

OK, now I was getting frustrated by not knowing which doctor was in charge of what here, and why I needed to see all of them. Anyhow, so I beg and probably whine a bit.

"Are you sure there is no way we can remove them today? They really hurt."

After all, it was not like he was incapable of removing them. I was qualified to remove them from an animal for crying out loud. So, bless his heart, he called my plastic surgeon and asked if it was OK for him to remove my tubes. Thankfully the go ahead was given. Yeah, relief was in sight.

Now, I had heard different things from different people in regard to what it felt like to remove the tubes. I had heard everything from "didn't hurt a bit," to "it's like pulling off a Band-Aid. Hurts, but by the time you yelp, it's over." So, I was figuring that the reaction of people had a lot to do with a combo of pain tolerance, and the amount of painkillers in their system when they had it done.   It turned out it also had a lot to do with how well you were healing.

The first thing the doctor asked me before snipping the sutures was "Did you bring your pain medicine with you?" No, but I had just taken them prior to coming to the appointment, so I should be good. Now, here was where I stop and caveat that I had been trying to reduce the amount of pain meds in order to not feel so sluggish. I had been dealing with some discomfort, but not any big deal. So, if you were like me and were trying that, I would give you this advice: Take your pain meds in full!

This hurt like crap. The first thing they did was snip the sutures, which felt like one more big tug on those already pulled hairs.

Ouch.

Then, they tell you to take a deep breath (not a good sign), and they do a quick yank to break the seal that has been created by your body as it healed and adhered to the tubes. Holy crap! Then they pulled out the tube, which was the funkiest feeling, as there was about a foot and a half of tubing up in there. What I had previously thought was the edge of my expander for reconstruction, was actually tubing, and you could feel it coming out. Guess what, that burned. Like fire. At least it did for me. I'm not saying everyone will hurt as bad as I did, but it hurt. It kind of felt like it ripped open everything in there again. Whoa.

Little did I know I was harboring an infection.

So, I went back on the full amount of pain meds, and now I was comfortable again, although sluggish. I wrote this in a relatively blissful fog and relatively pain free. Two steps forward, one step back. Oh well.

So, now the drains were out, which meant the fluids that had been draining now would accumulate in my body, and eventually be absorbed. No biggie. But the fluid was accumulating in my underarm, so when I put my arm down and squeeze, my boob (what was left of it) gains almost a cup size. When I release the pressure, I lose a cup size. It was kind of funny, really. If it wasn't uncomfortable to do, and if it didn't feel so weird, it would make a fun party trick. Of course, they may go in and drain this off today at my appointment with my plastic surgeon, but time would tell.

All this had been interesting, but I was so thankful for the fact that I had been complication and infection free throughout this process. This was especially a good thing as Alex had strep throat and impetigo (a skin infection in an open wound—highly contagious), and everyone seemed to have some mild tummy bug.

My house was filled with all these wonderful flowers, and cards, and foods, and love from so many people. It was wonderfully overwhelming! Just a year ago, I was in a real funk thinking those thoughts like if I died, would I be one of those people that no one would miss? Who would bother to come to my funeral? Would it be only five or ten? Or would I fill up the church? I was feeling like it would be the five or ten about this time last year. Last year was rough. I would still say rougher than this year so far. So the outpouring of love and prayer has really shown me an almost *It's a Wonderful Life* kind of awakening that I was loved. I could not thank everyone enough for that!

My prayer throughout this process had been that I would be cared for in my infirmity. I was used to being the one caring for others, not the one being cared for. That prayer has been answered ten-fold. I had been amazed and comforted by the amount of outpouring of love I had received. Thank you all. God works in the strangest ways. Strange and wonderful. This was a long road and a bit frustrating, in that I had no choice but to take it in His timing. But I was learning amazing lessons that He was teaching me. One of my friends said she could hardly wait to meet the woman I would become when this was over. Wow, the changes that I could feel happening in me through this were amazing. I was very curious what God would be doing with me once the lessons He had for me were learned.

And did I thank Lee in any of my "thank yous," of course not. Fool. Talk about denial! He had been fixing every meal, doing all the shopping and cleaning, and helping me take my medications, as I was not even strong enough to open the pill bottles. Yet, I was still so blindly mad, it meant nothing.

Missions

I'm hoping that I'm not being too optimistic in saying that I think I've finally turned that corner and was really feeling better. I've started to reduce the pain killers (again), and I do not hurt. I was a bit tender, but I do not hurt! I feel fabulous! My range of motion was slowly coming back, but I could now dress myself and brush my hair and teeth all by myself! Yeah! I could take a shower and wash my hair unassisted (OK, I couldn't dry it yet…). Although, I was still tired a lot, I felt more awake when I was awake. I could walk farther before getting tired.

Fred was home sick today. As with Alex when he was sick, he has been uncooperatively sequestered to his room (translation: he has to stay in his room and he didn't like it). It seems to be a different bug than what Alex had. I'm not sure if that was good or bad, I just didn't want it.

The sun was finally out. It felt like a lifetime since we had had real sunshine. It's even supposed to get up to sixty degrees today. What a concept! It was immensely healing to just sit in the sunshine, to soak up that sun with all its warmth, and promise. Then I would remember:

crap, I still have the BRCA2 gene, which causes skin cancer, and I had to wonder if I even needed sunscreen to sit in front of the window. I didn't know. It seemed really silly to slather on sunscreen all over just to spend an hour sitting in the sun in the window. Don't these windows filter out that type of light? I don't know. Which translates to: I better not sit in the sun without the sunscreen handy. Sigh.

> It was immensely healing to just sit in the sunshine.

I was amazed at how many previously simple things were now so complicated. I couldn't just sit in the sun. I couldn't go through menopause naturally. I'm not the type of person to choose to get plastic surgery, yet here I was getting my new set of breasts. I'm not the type to get tattoos, yet I'll be getting at least two. I'm not upset, mind you; just observing all the stuff that didn't go "as planned."

I think one of my most favorite movie scenes has to be from *Evan Almighty*, where the main character, "Evan," (played by Steve Carell), was talking to "God," (played by Morgan Freeman). Evan tells God that he has plans, and God looks at him says, "Oh, you have plans?" and then just laughs. I love that scene because it really epitomizes (gee, I must be feeling better, I'm using lots of big words here) the fact that no matter what we think our plans are or should be, God has other plans, and His plans will always be more important than our plans. This was the perfect opportunity to sit, and listen to what He would have me do. He has taken away all other distractions during this time of healing.

I was listening to what God wanted me to do, huh? Well, although that was true, I decided to ignore what He was telling me about my marriage. I pointedly ignored everything Lee was doing for me in order to retain being angry, done, ready to move out and move on, all the while thinking I was in my right to feel this way. Lee had taken several weeks off of work, drove me to every single appointment, and took care of my every need. Did I give him even a shred of credit? Of course not. I felt like he owed it to me. I felt like he had let me down so completely that I deserved this; he owed me this much (not that it made anything any better). So instead of giving him credit to prove he was a good husband, while the other times had been poor spousal moments, I still felt angry and resentful about all that had transpired and steadfastly believed he was a bad husband.

Our church made a wonderful announcement a few weeks ago. We had a surplus of funds in our missions fund. So much so that we needed to find out how the church should spend it. So the church asked us "What is YOUR mission?" Wow, what a question. What was my mission? What was my mission as I sit here typing, still unable to lift ten pounds, unable to drive (painkillers), and not cognizant enough to be able to coordinate anything? So many of my "dreams" or ideas for missions had frittered away due to reality checks, physical inability (sorry, but I couldn't throw around fifty pounds anymore, so it would not be likely I could really work at the zoo), timing, or God letting me know that this was not a good idea.

I hope to feel like a phoenix reborn in a way, with renewed purpose when I was better. For now, I got to concentrate on other things, like shaving.

I was numb in my arm pits. No feeling. Probably won't ever get it back. I don't mind, but it created a really interesting situation when it came to shaving and putting on deodorant. As any woman who shaves knows, shaving the arm pits was a very tender procedure. If you scrape too hard with the razor, you get razor burn. Guys know about razor burn. However, they do not know about how fun it is to have razor burn and then sweat. It hurts, it stings, it causes irritation that hurts like crazy and can get infected rather easily. Joy. OK, so now, throw in that you cannot feel how hard you are pressing. I may not feel it, but I may have just shaved off the first three layers of skin and not know it. Joy. They should come out with a new deodorant for women in my condition that contains Neosporin®, just to be on the safe side. When I put on deodorant, or shaved, it felt like I was rubbing through clothing, as if I had on a shirt and was trying to shave through the shirt. What a bizarre feeling that was.   I could see I missed a few spots, but at least I did not have a doctor appointment today.

Well, ladies and germs, the meds were working, and my head was getting fuzzy, so I went back to bed. Our purpose in life may be different than what we think. What do you think yours is? Maybe you need to ask "What is His mission for me?"

The Reasons Why

I find it interesting, all the little things that you find out during the process of a surgery like mine, where when you discover the reasons for some of the things you were told to do, you suddenly go "Oh, now I get it!" I had the privilege of finding some awesome articles that gave some fabulous tips of what to do before my surgery, which I heeded and followed. They all were spot on. I did not, however, understand the reasons for all of them. To me, understanding the why was as important as the do.

Buy 5 extra pillows, and at least 2 body pillows.

OK, why? Well, because after surgery you would be very sore, and could only sleep on your back for weeks to months (if you were having reconstruction), and I guarantee that you will need all those pillows behind your back, under your knees, and also padded behind you, so that you could have the privilege of sleeping slightly propped on your side which, after a month of sleeping only on your back, feels like heaven.

Then there were the safety pins. You didn't need many, just two to three large safety pins (depending on how many drains you got). If you could find just a few safety pins or just took a few from your sewing kit (if you had one), do so, or buying a pack was not expensive.

OK, why? Well, the drainage tubes you have coming out of you are a bit unruly, long (about two and a half feet), and they pull like crazy to come out. Pinning them up helps to keep them under your clothes, so it's not as embarrassing to walk about. It also keeps them from pulling so hard, and it makes it much easier to go potty because when you sit, you tend to bump the tubes, which in turn bumps the areas that they go into your body, which hurts. Along this road, I met a fabulous gal who has designed some shirts and aprons to hold the nasty drains in little pockets inside the shirt (apron) and help you to feel more comfortable. Her company is called "Heal In Comfort." Check them out. She's a breast cancer veteran, too.

Camisoles and sports bras. Buy a bunch.

OK, why? This one I did not understand until my Doctor told me at my last appointment when I asked. I wish I would have understood the reason prior to buying the ones I did, because now I had to buy more. I figured that I needed to wear these, since I could not wear a regular bra until everything was complete. Well, although that was partly true in the early stages, the reasons were different and very important. When they take the Steri-strips off (the tape they would put over the sutures), the sutures were not necessarily immediately removed. They leave them in for quite a while as you heal, to make sure you are really well healed before they start expansion. Until then, the sutures and your incision sites are subject to constant rubbing by movement of your clothing. So they want you to have a good sports bra (after you are cleared to lift your arms above your head), or camisole with shelf bra, so that the general movement of life isn't constantly rubbing the incisions. I ended up using tank tops more than anything else, as they were the most comfortable for me.

Pain meds. DO NOT get behind on your pain meds! A schedule will appear; stick to it!

OK, why? If you skip a dose or two (especially in the early days), the pain comes on as if you had the surgery without any meds at all. It's excruciating! Make sure even the nurses stick to this! The young nurses had often not learned this yet. I had a young nurse who let me sleep past time to take meds, and I was in a lot of pain by the time I woke up. My husband, bless his heart, thought I was sleeping so peacefully the first night I got home that he let me sleep, and I missed two doses. I woke up screaming in pain. It took more than twelve hours to start to feel better and get the pain under control again. Not a good day. I cannot emphasize this enough. Keep up with the schedule. Have someone help you get your meds in the night. You may not even have the strength in your upper body to open the medicine bottles, not even the easy-open ones. The thing you need to realize is that some people are not able to get back in control of the pain if doses are missed, and they have to spend days or weeks in pain, while taking the maximum dosages of meds, just because they got "behind the pain" once. Stay comfortable, lose a tad bit of sleep, take the meds ON TIME!

Electric toothbrush.

OK, why? I read this in an article. I already had one, so was not concerned until the first time I brushed my teeth. You need to understand that when they put in implants, they mess with muscle tissue. In a way, they strain all your chest muscles. Ever pull a muscle really bad? It hurts. Not only that, you kind of can't use it for a while, right? Well, that was essentially what was happening here. Translation: You have NO upper body strength. You cannot sit up unassisted, you cannot pull your pants up and down to go potty unassisted, and you cannot make the back and forth motion to brush your teeth for the amount of time needed to actually brush properly. You are going to feel dirty, tired, and totally drugged out. Any little thing to help out for now would seem like a God-send.

Sweat pants.

OK, why? Pretty simple here. We are going for comfort and ease. As stated, at first, you can't even pull your own pants up and down. Get a couple of pairs. Be prepared to have to go out in public in them (mostly to doctors' appointments), for lack of being comfortable in anything else. Forgot the fashion factor here ladies, comfort is the word of the day!

Button-down shirts in soft material.

OK, why? Now, the thing with button-down shirts was that, again, comfort was key here. You are not allowed to lift your arms, and it hurts to even try. I bought a ton of wonderful second-hand button-down shirts in a fabulous material that I now could not wear. Why? Some of the shirts I could not wear because my arms swelled up too much to fit, and others because the nerves were so raw for a time that I could not wear specific materials. Silky-type materials felt horrible. They just plain hurt. For me, anything along the lines of fluffy and soft (my bathrobe) felt very comfortable. Now, I do not know if this is true for everyone, but the rawness of my nerves created an issue with how I chose to dress myself every day. Even now, almost a month later, this was true. The nerves were getting much better. Some of the nerves were becoming totally numb, others were regaining feeling. I knew it would be months until they calmed down. Just expect it.

Slip on Shoes.

OK, why? Because you were not going to be able to reach your feet for a while. You will not have the reach. Along with the straining feeling of the muscles, you will feel tied up, as if something was preventing you from fully extending your arms, and if you try... well, I do not recommend it unless you are into pain. You will not be able to tie your shoes either for a time. Of course, if you have someone who will constantly be available to do this for you, well, OK then. However, if you plan on being relatively self-sufficient, you will need slip-ons. I still could not pull on shoes and tie them for over a month after surgery.

Keep a pillow in the car.

OK, why? Because the seatbelt right across your chest will be terribly painful, and you don't even want to think about how much pain you will be in if you have a short stop for any reason. I found that just going over bumps on the road were painful. You will not be in the car much at first, but then again, you will not want to go anywhere for a bit. You will not be allowed to drive until you are off all your pain meds. Most of them are narcotics and make you sleepy. Besides, you don't want to have to be driving with a pillow strapped to the front of you anyhow.

Ah, one more note: transportation. You will not be able to pull yourself up into a truck or SUV. You will not have the strength to open and shut the car doors. If you have a really low sitting car, you may have a bit of trouble getting in and out of that, too.   It will get better, but it will be a pain for a while.

That's all I could think of off the top of my head. I'm sure there will be more.

Yes, none of this is for the faint of heart, but it was such a small price to pay for knowing I could watch my boys finish growing up. It's a small price to pay for knowing in the end, I shouldn't have to have breast cancer ever again. It's a small price to pay in knowing that I would get to yet again try to make a garden grow, and raise more orphaned kittens, and in short, enjoy life. So take heart. Keep a stiff upper lip, and just do the next thing.

Home Again
(Smackdown)

OK, here is where I add in the all-important God moment that happened Saturday night. I felt like Lee was not taking as good of care of me as I felt I needed. I felt as if he was starting to slip, and I decided to talk to him about it. Well, chew him out was a bit closer to the mark, I think. I told him that he needed to step it up a bit, because I was worried that he had become complacent. I was worried that if something happened and I needed him fast that I would get a "in a minute" which would translate to an "I'll get there when I feel like it."

So, I explained to him that I was not out of the woods yet as far as getting an infection, and that they come on in the blink of an eye. I wanted him to understand that if I got sick at say, 0200 (that was two in the morning), and asked him to take me to the hospital, a response of "in the morning" was not going to be acceptable. That conversation was a 2200 Saturday night and lasted until 2300 Saturday night. Guess what happened at 0100 Sunday? Well, I could never seem to do things the easy way, no matter how hard I tried, or with the best intentions. All I could say was I followed my doctor's instructions to the best of my ability, but still got a raging secondary infection in the middle of the night. At 0100 I woke up with chills, body aches, and all the signs of a fever. When I took my temperature at 0230, it was normal. However, still feeling horrible, I took my temp again at 0330, this time I had a one hundred and one point five degree temperature. Time for me to go to the hospital. Joy. Gee, do you think I was getting a very strong comment from God here? Maybe just a bit. And how did I react? I wasn't sure if the lesson was for me or for Lee. I will admit, it was for both of us, but I think the timing of it was just for me.

The first question to answer was what had caused this fever? It could be the flu. It could be a post-operative infection. It could be something else entirely. So, then the fun began of testing and trying to determine why I was having these issues. After several hours, we still had not come to a definite conclusion. What we did know was that I was very sick.

One thing to note for those of you who have never experienced invasive surgery in your own life, or have never walked with someone through it, is to know that secondary infections tend to happen in the blink of an eye, and get really bad, really fast. The doctors aren't kidding when they tell you to call if you have a fever, even a little one. Even if you are just feeling a bit under the weather, start paying attention so you can catch it early.

So, I knew now that I had an infection of the left side. I was so swollen that I looked about the size I used to be before my mastectomy. I should say here that I had underestimated the amount of pain I was in. I hurt so badly that every time the doctor tried to listen to my heart, I practically screamed in pain. I neglected to take this as a sign that something was wrong. Granted, it hurt, and I knew this was a bad thing, but it was also a reminder of why I was bothering with this road. That reminder was important right now, because if we could not get this infection to clear up then I had to go back into surgery, where they would remove the implants (maybe on both sides), clean out the wounds, and then decide if they could put in new ones.

Now, let me explain the "if" in that last sentence. The "if" meant there were some things that may be going on. One possibility was that I had to heal first without the implants, and then go back in and to have them put in fresh implants. The second "if" pertained to the very real possibility that this infection was a rejection type issue, and I may not be a candidate for reconstruction after all. Time would tell.

So, for now I was home (YEAH!) and I had in a PICC (Peripherally Inserted Central Catheter) line, which was basically a type of IV line that was longer lasting and a ton more comfortable. It was inserted just above the elbow on the inner arm. They feed the line into a major vein and end up just above the top of the heart. Once they put in the catheter, there were about four inches left dangling outside you for the caps, where you attach and detach the IV lines. That way you were not hooked up twenty-four hours a day and could have more mobility. These tubes were held in place by a type of tape that was clear where the insertion point was, so you could observe for infection. My body didn't like this stuff, but I did not get a choice. Neither did my skin. Time would tell how my skin reacted with my tape sensitivity.

I had a portable at-home IV machine that delivered my medications. I could not do all of the hooking up and unhooking by myself, and there was a level of sterility needed, as well as being sure you were not adding air into your lines. It was a bit scary, but you adapt. I had a nurse come and teach my hubby and me how to properly and safely do everything.

I'm actually starting to hurt less (the pain I had been in was also a sign of an infection, mind you!), and was taking almost half of the pain meds I was before going into the hospital. I had all sorts of fun equipment at home now, because I had to get hooked up to an IV pump about four times a day for heavy-duty antibiotics. Hey, I'll take it, I'm home and I feel better.

The flip side was that I had been having issues with not enough trips to the potty, thanks to the pain meds, and now I was having too many trips to the potty, thanks to the antibiotics. Ah, the joy in understanding how the body works was sometimes a little head-shaking in disbelief. But, this too shall pass, and pass, and pass.

Dresses

It was a simple, honest question. Was I interested in going to the military formal ball in April? I knew he asked because, previously, had he not asked, I would have come unglued. I love the formal balls! They were a wonderful excuse to dress up like a princess, treat yourself to getting your hair and nails done, and buy and wear expensive jewelry. And then there was the dress. Oh, the dress. I had the best dress. The type of dress that snaps heads. OK, I know I was being stared at because of the dress more than me being in it, but still, the effect was flattering nonetheless.

I bought the dress on my most successful shopping trip in Seoul when we lived in Korea. In Korea (yes, South Korea), they haggle over buying things. To me, this was so confrontational, and I never could quite get the gist of it, and whether I had ticked off or impressed the sales ladies. Often, it was both. I was no good.

Now, in Korea, the women are very slim by comparison here, and at a size twelve, I was at the very top weight that they considered socially acceptable, while still having clothes that fit in the regular stores. So shopping could be really interesting sometimes. In this store, which had formals, I was really struggling to find anything that fit.

Finally, the sales lady brings out this jaw dropping, unbelievably gorgeous, looks like a dress for the fabulously rich, dress. It was a gorgeous color of teal, and made of satin. The entire dress was hand sewn and hand beaded with iridescent beads, not sequins; beads. If this dress was for sale in the USA, it easily would have been over $2,000. In this shop, it was just $700. That was still more than I could handle. It fit like a glove, and was phenomenal! I actually (with a long cool story attached to it) got the dress for $325!

Did I want to go to the Military Ball? It was a simple question that brought me to tears. The dress, THE dress, was strapless, and backless. In my current state, I couldn't wear it. No way. I could barely wear regular clothes yet, much less a potentially uncomfortable dress (mine was not). No way could I go to the ball. Anyone seen my fairy godmother handy?

You see, it was, in the end, *that* dress that made me decide to get implants. I knew that if I didn't I could never wear that dress again. I wanted to wear that dress again, at least one more time.

I remind myself that it was only for now. This time next year, hopefully, I could wear that dress again. It was part of my healing. There was still emotional healing going on with it all, too. I guess I was not quite there yet. Either way, I had to pass on going to this ball. I would (oddly enough) almost prefer to go bald than breastless to a ball. With hair loss, at least it's obvious you've been ill. Upon outward appearance I do not look ill, save for the current pasty complexion, and PICC line hanging out of my arm. Formal dresses were often preformed so that you could forego a bra, and therefore part of the fit was filling out the bodice of the dress. Others were really clingy and sometimes along the lines of still going without a bra (think the really slinky dresses here).

Either way, I was out of luck. Add to that I had the issue of the pain involved in anything rubbing up against and irritating my sutures still. I just couldn't bring myself go to a formal ball in a cotton camisole and zip-front hoody sweatshirt. That was OK. It was for now. But right now, I was feeling rather jealous of Cinderella.

Seromas and Flowers

I suppose a writing like this would be very boring to read if everything went smoothly. Yeah, we'll go with that. I had successfully had what you would call major complications. (Successfully? Like I tried?) I think things had been off since the first surgery on February twenty fifth. I was in terrible pain from the beginning. I didn't get better, at least not by much. They put me on antibiotics for two weeks, right out of surgery. During that time, I got the tubes out and remained in a lot of pain. I was amazed at how much pain I was in. But, I soldiered on. I figured that was normal. I was convinced it would get better. Then I got the fever. OK. I went into the hospital, and I had an infection. A nasty one. While I was in the hospital at the end of March, the left side swelled up, and I got a hot red spot on one side. I was put on strong antibiotics and sent home a day later. I was still in pain, but less pain than before by quite a bit. However, the swelling continued, and the red spot got bigger and hotter. I was told to wait for the antibiotics to work.

By now, I was caught between throwing a fit and yelling something was wrong, fix it, and trying to trust my doctors as I continued to get sicker. On Friday, a week ago, I went back in to see my doctor. He drew a "line in the sand," meaning he drew lines around the red spot and said if it got any worse, I should go to the hospital. Although it didn't get any bigger, I ended up in the hospital anyway. Why? Because I couldn't breathe.

I felt like someone was pushing on my chest, but only on the left side where the swelling was. It didn't hurt; I just couldn't take a deep breath. Boy, did the ER jump when I came in and said I couldn't breathe! Good thing too, ideally. A lot could go very wrong very fast when you can't breathe. All the oxygen machines in the hospital said I was getting enough oxygen for my body, but I just couldn't breathe deeply.

I tell you what though, I was very glad I had in my PICC line, because they didn't have to put in an IV. Yeah!

Boy that sounds warped.

Basically what was going on was that I was so swollen, with so much fluid in the left side, it was pushing in, because it had pushed out as far as it could. To give you an idea, I looked like my expansion was done and I had the new implant in. I even teased the doctor that he had put in new expanders that were remotely activated.

So, back into the hospital I went. They put me on even stronger antibiotics. This type, called Vancomycin, was some of the big guns. This stuff could only be given in a PICC line because it was so hard on the veins that you couldn't give it "just" in the IV line. Whoa. I was one sick puppy. It was weird because I didn't really hurt by comparison to how badly I had been hurting already from the surgery. I wasn't as fuzzy as I had felt in weeks previous. I was able to get up, move around, go to the bathroom unassisted (a biggie in the hospital), but I was SICK. Great.

By Monday morning it was obvious they were going to have to do surgery again. I was originally scheduled for 1000 surgery Monday morning. That was changed to 1700 by Monday morning, and at 1245 I was informed that surgery was changed again to 1300 because they had a cancellation of another surgery. Here we go! At least I was ready and had not eaten, so it was fast and smooth.

The surgery didn't last long. They went in, cleaned me out, removed bit of infected tissue, the expanders were replaced, and then I was stitched back up.

It turned out that not only did I have a ton of fluid, but had developed a seroma. A seroma was basically a blob of coagulated blood stuff. Kind of like a scab that develops under the skin. That's a poor explanation, but it was good enough for now.

Because of that seroma, I would not have gotten better without getting it removed. They also put in another drainage tube. Yeah, my favorite. Oh well, this would keep another seroma from developing. I'll deal.

I had to say that I felt better after surgery, for the most part, than before I went in. That was always a good thing. I was now on less meds, in less pain, more comfortable, and still on the knockout antibiotics. I was officially still fighting this infection. I'd like to say I was winning, but I would be very guarded in my optimism, simply because I was feeling a bit discouraged.

Would this all have happened if I would have foregone the implants? Was I going to get better now? Did I have more ahead? I didn't dare ask "what next?" I was not sure I wanted to know, unless it was that I would finally get better. I was originally planning on getting my other big surgery, the oophorectomy, done towards the end of April. Screw that. Right now I didn't want to have to have more surgery for a long time. I decided I would have my oophorectomy and the putting-in of the final implants done at the same time. I was tired of all this. I know some people have problems with their implants that last for years. I did wonder, in the back of my mind, would I be one of them?

Then I figured if I ended up having them removed and going with prosthetics, I could throw my boobs at my doctor, That made me smile, and I felt better.

I forgot to mention that I got my stitches out on my right side. They took them out during surgery on the left side. It's a wicked scar, but looks good, really. I was supposed to get some vitamin E to rub (LIGHTLY) on the incision to lessen the scar. That side looks bumpy because of the expander, which was more visible since the swelling was gone on that side. I was, as of now, home and in remarkably less pain than I had been in over a month. For that I was grateful. I was achy, but no sharp pains. I was still weak, and was going to stay that way for the moment, but that was OK. I was learning my limits, and schedules. I was on the antibiotics that required me to hook myself up, (with help) to the IV pump through my PICC line and get a dose of the powerhouse antibiotics twice a day for about an hour. No biggie. I had this done once in the morning, and once in the evening. I got to sleep through the night! How cool was that? Haven't done that in over a month! I woke up without being in a ton of pain. I also got a home nurse that came in occasionally and helped me with the PICC line. She was really nice, and we got along well.

This infection and surgery were real turning points in many ways. First off, I realized that I really was in excruciating pain. I knew it would hurt, and I thought the level of pain I was in was normal. I was wrong. I was in terrible pain because I had an infection. We had no idea when the infection may have started, but it was definitely before the initial removal of the original set of drainage tubes.

The other major turning point was the PICC line. As I mentioned, I needed help. Who do you think helped me? Well, my home nurse, of course. She came in a few times a week and helped me change the dressings and make sure everything was going as planned. Or at least that was what I told people. The fact was that something huge was happening with my relationship with Lee. When you were being hooked up to IV meds, there was a true margin of error there. He could have screwed up, not gotten all the air out of the lines, and he could have made me more sick. I was not in a position to do it myself, and half the time I was so drugged up that I was not conscious while he administered the meds. I literally had to put my life one hundred percent in his hands and trust he would take care of me, and that I would be safe.

Let me set the stage a bit more for you … There were two IV lines hanging out of my arm that had to be alternated, so one does not clog up. The process starts by cleaning the connections, hooking up the bag of meds to the machine, and bleeding the air out of the IV tube, all before hooking it up to the tubes in my arm. First, he made sure the line we had to use was still open by giving a push of saline. Then, he hooked up the lines to me, turned on the machine, and then we would wait until the meds were done. At that point, he would disconnect me from the meds and give me another push of saline to make sure I got the entire intended dose of medication, (which, by the way, was kept in the refrigerator). At that point, I was disconnected from the machine. Then, to make sure the line did not clog up between doses, he added a push of heparin, which was a medication to keep the blood from clotting.

I literally had to put my life one hundred percent in his hands and trust he would take care of me.

Now, there were several important points in here; several places that, if things were done wrong, could cause complications. If Lee mixed up the heparin and the saline, that would have been bad. People die from those types of mistakes. If he had not bled the lines of the air, that would have been bad: Yet another error with potentially fatal consequences. If the doses were not given at the right time, that would have allowed the infection to learn to fight the antibiotics. There was lots of room for error here. This procedure, which lasted about 35-40 minutes, was performed around the clock. At first, I needed the meds every 6 hours, which meant there was going to be a dose in the middle of the night. So poor Lee had to get up in the middle of the night and be coherent enough to go through this process for me every night, for weeks. He never once complained. He did awesomely. I had to put my life completely in his hands, and he did a beautiful job. Yet, I remained steadfastly set on being mad at him.

Who of you, on the brink of divorce, would allow your soon-to-be-ex anywhere near you with that sort of situation? Certainly not many. I was too sick to have a choice. However, I have to say, he did an unbelievably wonderful job. His attention to detail was well above reproach, and he did amazing, especially considering anything like this usually makes him queasy and almost pass out.

With the new drain in, I was back to not being able to take a shower or bath. Bummer. To me I constantly felt dirty, like I couldn't get the stinkiness of body odor off of me. Oh well, that's what perfume is for, isn't it? Washing my hair was quite a trial, but we muddled through. I almost wanted to hack off my hair for ease of washing, but it took me two years to grow it this long, and I didn't want to wait another two to grow it back. Besides, it was only for a while.

It was finally spring, glorious spring! I could open the windows and listen to the birds, feel the warmth of the sunshine, and go outside without freezing my fanny off. I looked at my poor little gardens and all I planned to do with them this year. Oh well. We'll just let God handle the gardens this year. He was in control anyhow. That reality helped. I knew there was a reason I was going through all these tribulations with my surgeries. Life looks different than it did three months ago. It's shifting, changing, in fast, dramatic ways. If I wasn't in the midst of it, I would kind of like to just sit back and watch and analyze it all.

For now, I would settle for watching the leaves come in on the trees and the flowers bloom around me. And heal.

He is Risen

"He is risen!" He was risen, indeed! Yup, it's Easter. No, I didn't make it to church. That just feels wrong, but I had come to the realization that I needed to stay down and house bound for now and heal, really heal. I admit I thought I was doing better, but how many times had I said that already? I'll let the doc tell me I'm better first this time.

I had greater use of my right arm and hand now as opposed to the last surgery, and for that I was grateful. I could move easier, dress easier, eat easier, and groom easier. I already had more ease of movement in the left arm than I did even two weeks ago. This was good. But I was far from one hundred percent.

As I became more comfortable, and actually healed, there were all sorts of little "ah-ha" moments that made sense in hint sight. One of the biggest was how to care for the drainage tube hanging out of my body. I finally, out of curiosity, measured it. It was 3 feet long, and that was what was just on the outside of my body. As you may recall, I felt like it was being ripped out of my body last time, and

I was so miserable with it. Every movement seemed to make it hurt. This time was a totally different story. This time, I was comfortable, it didn't pull, and I did not bump it nearly as badly. I did things a bit differently this time. Consequently, I wanted to write these tips down, in case I ever needed to have these again, and in case anyone else might find them useful.

You needed to safety pin them to your clothing. You couldn't let it dangle, and to be honest, you wouldn't want it to anyhow, because that would really hurt. Last time, I had one safety pin that pinned the end of the tube to the opposite side of my body. The tube came out of the left side, and I pinned it to the right. I found that I bumped it every time I walked, sat, and sometimes caught it with my hands as I moved. It wasn't very stable. This time, I pinned it to the opposite side of my body about half way up the tube. And then I looped it back again to pin the end back below where it comes out of my body. As long as you keep those pins below the level of the drain, it works. It was more stable, and I didn't bump it nearly as much. At home I would pin them on the outside of my clothes for my own comfort, and no one in the house cared. When I went out, I pinned them inside of my clothes.

But that change alone was still not quite enough to make it comfortably stable. The final to do was to take a piece of tape or two, and tape the tube down about 2-3 inches below where it comes out of my body. That reduced the amount of pulling directly against the tube. That was probably the biggest thing I did to provide myself comfort. Now, for me this was a tradeoff. I was sensitive to the adhesives on tape. They make me itch and could cause a rash. It was a lesser of two evils kind of thing for me. But boy, was I glad I did it. My comfort level was night and day. By two weeks post-surgery last time, I was miserable. This time, when I went in to see my doctor, if he told me I needed to have the drain in another week, instead of crying (which I totally would have done last time), I could say, "sure, no problem." Do note that I did have the infections going last time. I did not know how much that really affected the pain levels.

Remember the icky leaking? It was still an issue. Last time I used maxi pads. This time I decided that was not the best idea for two reasons. Number one was that I didn't leak nearly enough to need that much absorption, at least not if you were healing well. The second was that I think the thickness of the pad pulled at the tubes and caused some of the discomfort. This time I took some rolled gauze, cut about three to four inches, folded it in quarters, and very carefully slipped it under the tube. The bottom of the gauze would sit just about at the top of the tape, so you could tape it down just at the top of the tape/bottom of the gauze. This worked great, and was much more comfortable. If I found I was still getting drips on my clothing, I could put a Band-Aid lightly over the top where it leaked, but that didn't happen enough this time to be necessary.

Even the critters in the house do their part. The cats never leave my side; neither does Bud, the dog. I was heartened by the birds singing both inside and out and the smell of fresh air as the weather warmed. Around here, with the wind coming from the south, the "fresh smell" was cow, but, hey, I'll take it.

So many people talk about how their pets help them get better. It's true. They are content to just sit with you for hours and hours. They don't mind what tubes are coming out of you. They don't mind if you are grumpy or crying. All they know is that you are hurting, and they wanted to be there to take care of you as best they could. I loved them.

They also provided a huge source of enjoyment and laughter. That morning our kitten, which had had his own rough road with a spinal injury, was curled up on the bed beside my hubby. He (the kitten) lazily looked up at us with his hysterically crossed eyes (I really shouldn't laugh, because they were that way from a head injury we think, but it's so cute), and his little tongue sticking out at us. He truly looked like he was trying to make faces at us, but the fact that he was oblivious to our laughter made it even funnier. We did manage to grab a camera and got a shot or two, but the pictures weren't nearly as funny as being there.

The leaves were coming out on the trees. I love watching them. This week would be huge because this was about the time they suddenly pop. They just started on my dad's birthday, which just passed, and they were usually pretty full on the trees only a week later, by my hubby's birthday. Spring was such a wonderful time to heal. There was so much beauty around in the world that really helped to lift the spirit. I took a short walk yesterday, the first one since my second surgery. It felt great. Hopefully now I could start walking and really enjoy the spring!

Femininity or Lack Thereof

I was entitled to a day where I was frustrated, discouraged, and in general moody, right? I got that just for being female, really, so this should be a non-issue. However, I had to admit, today was starting off awfully low. Although I was taking much less pain medication, and things were functioning more normally, there was a flip side. It really may be a little too soon to put the meds away. I was achy and just uncomfortable enough, (but not "hurting") that I felt yucky. I haven't slept in two days, because I couldn't get comfortable enough to fall asleep.

I did see my doctors yesterday, and they were happy with my current progress, however, when the blood tests came in they increased my antibiotics. I was healing, I was feeling better, but I was not there yet. Maybe I would in another week. I was OK with that.

No, I'm lying. I was tired of being sick and tired. I was so thrilled to have found my cancer so early that I could forego chemo and radiation: I was going to have a relatively short "illness" period, and be up and about in less than a month. So much for that.

So, I conceded that even though I did not hurt, the achiness was too much to forego pain meds all together. Two steps forward, one step back. I wondered often if I would be having the same complications if I was not doing reconstruction. Would I have chosen to go that route had I known I was going to have this much trouble? How many more complications were ahead? After all, I was committed to this course of action now. The implant expanders were in. If I changed my mind, I had to have more surgery. If I proceeded, I still had to have more surgery. Right now, I was really rethinking the idea of nipple reconstruction. Did I really need to go to that length to feel "normal enough" to feel female? Would just tattooing be enough? At least I did not have to make that decision yet. I was not happy about the idea of possible complications with the implants further down the road (leaks and ruptures).

I wanted to feel well enough to go dancing. Actually, I would settle for feeling well enough to go out to dinner. Even feeling well enough to put on "real clothes" (translate into looks nice, feels nice) would be a plus. The nerve pain was almost all gone, which was fabulous, but there was still a patch under my right arm that was sensitive to materials, and so I had to be picky with what I wore. And by picky, I mean it needed to be extra soft and fluffy to feel good; nothing clingy, or silky, or smooth. Not even drapey. So lots of flannel and fleece, and the best thing was still my bathrobe. Now that the spring had begun, I needed to find soft warm-weather things to wear. I was praying that I would feel better enough by the time that became a real issue. Then again, as much time as I was stuck in the house right now, it really didn't matter.

Beating the cancer was easy. I would admit the assault on my femininity has been harder than expected. Maybe it was because I never really did feel very feminine, and now I didn't look it either. I heard so many women who haven't gone through this say they would pass on reconstruction, because they were not attached enough to their breasts. I knew more friends that did not get reconstruction who said they were more happy with how they look now, than those who got reconstruction. I suppose that they were more comfortable with their femininity. I didn't know. I grew up with a cancer veteran who did not have reconstruction. It's not like I didn't know what it was all about. It wasn't like I thought my mom should have gotten reconstruction. She was not a candidate. Either way, it was something normal for me. I guess that was why I was having trouble understanding why this was such a struggle.

I sat and looked at my budding garden and all the weeds coming up that I wished I had the strength to pull. My garden was going to be absolutely unruly this year (OK, it usually was, but I was really planning stuff with it this year). Usually, I could get all the dead stuff pulled up and cleaned up, and pull some of the weeds. Not this year. The boys hate to garden, and getting them to help was like pulling teeth. So, I guess I got to just sit back and let whatever comes up, come.

I wanted to look ahead and plan something, even just a trip, but felt like I could not. I wanted to plan something fun, but I was too unsure, too frustrated. Too tired of having to change and cancel the plans I did make.

One day at a time.

Keep the faith, keep the hope.

Roll with the punches.

Get back up on that horse.

Yeah, I know, but for the moment, pardon me while I indulge myself by wallowing in self-pity for the day. And figure out how to deal with the phantom itch I had where my right breast used to be.

Genes and Toys

I woke up this morning with a surge of energy and a great outlook. I love mornings like this: Mornings that you look at the sun coming through the window and go "BRING IT ON!" and feel like you could take on the world. The feeling may not last, I may get to lunch time and be snoozing on the couch, but it did my heart good to feel generally optimistic about the world.

OK, I really want to make a plea to all my loved ones here: GET GENETIC TESTING FOR CANCER! I understand how so many of you don't want to know, as if the results were a death sentence or date to die. I want you to think of it a different way.

What if you were told (convinced, prophesied, whatever) that you would be in a car accident at Second Street and Main in your city? No date, nothing about the outcome of the accident, just that you would be having one *there*. Would you want to know? I would. Because there was something I could do to avoid it.

Second and Main? I would be taking different routes from then on, or maybe beefing up my driving skills. You better believe I'd be getting a safer car! Now, what if there were several members of your family who also got into car accidents at that same intersection? Wouldn't you change what you were doing so you didn't have to have an accident, too? Would you have preferred that Toyota not had the recall and those brake failures be deemed an unfortunate hazard of driving a car? How many of you have Toyotas? Did you take yours in to get looked at or were you sitting in your car and praying yours in not going to have brake problems too? The genetic testing is like the recall. Find out if you are even at a high risk.

To me, that was what the genetic testing for cancer meant. It told me if I needed a plan. Because, people, there are options! This isn't like you get the diagnosis and wait to die or something. You **You can be proactive!** can be proactive! Insurance can no longer consider you to have a pre-existing condition if you get the testing done, and the results are positive for cancer genes. Plus, by getting the testing, you can argue with the insurance companies for how much cheaper and healthier preventable measures would be as opposed to getting cancer and then cancer treatments. That is what I did.

The BRCA2 gene, the one I have, was responsible for three cancers: breast, ovarian, and skin. It is triggered into action by estrogen hormones: caused in part by estrogen. People: we have a cause (one of, but not the only) for these cancers! Now we could do something. There are meds to reduce the risks of your getting cancer. There are lifestyle changes that would definitely reduce your risks. There are simple surgeries to reduce your risks by up to 86%.   Are you really willing to do nothing but sit back and wait and wonder?

Cancer is hell. You get sick, and complications are magnified a million times, not to mention the stress on your body and the toll it takes on your family. Wouldn't you like to take steps to avoid it if you could? That's what the testing could do for you!

I've always known I would get this. It was always just a matter of when. I found my cancer blessedly early, and now I would not be getting breast cancer again. Yes, I would have preferred to just have had removed the ovaries and kept the breasts. It didn't work out that way for me, but maybe it could for you.

To the men in my life: GET TESTED, TOO! You are still at risk. No, you can't have your ovaries removed, but there are medications that you guys can take to reduce your risks of breast cancer and skin cancer. Yes, men can get breast cancer! Prostate cancer is in the same family of cancers, there may now be meds for that, too.

I hate the idea of throwing a pill at every problem, or even have "elective" surgeries. However, since I knew I was going to get cancer, I did what it took. I wish you would too! I love you, and I want you to be healthy, and strong, and cancer free. Cancer is a nasty foe. One I would rather kick to the curb before it bites me.

OK. Lecture over.

I do wish to tell you a story that happened yesterday. It's a shameless plug to encourage you to train your dogs well, because you never knew when they, or you, might really be in a situation where they need to mind unquestioningly.

My dog, Bud, a Golden Retriever, is awesome and very well behaved. He loves to carry things in his mouth at all times, usually shoes or a stuffed animal. He never chews the shoes and rarely chews up his stuffed animals. But he was obsessive compulsive about having them in his mouth at all times. When he goes out to go potty, we make him leave his toys in the house because dog-slobbered stuffed animals left out in the rain smell particularly bad in the house. Consequently, when he comes back in he usually runs straight to his nearest toy, grabs it quick and makes a victory lap or two around the house, running with wild abandon.

Well, yesterday, I did something a bit out of my norm by bringing my IV pump down from my bedroom to the living room because some friends and my nurse came over, and I just didn't want to have everyone in my bedroom. The pump has a battery, and so I set it on the table by my favorite chair and got all plugged in. About half way through the one-hour session, I was alone again, and Bud needed to go out to go potty. No problem. My IV cord reaches about six feet, and so I got up to let him out. When he was done, I let him in.

Right after I let him in, I turned just in time to see that my IV cord was nicely draped over his favorite and closest toy. In the blink of an eye Bud was snatching up his toy, and my IV line, in his mouth, and just about to run his victory lap. Holy cow. Remember, I had a PICC line which was a catheter going from my elbow up to the top of my heart, and I guarantee that having it violently yanked out would not have been a good thing. Neither would the cost of replacing the IV pump, which no doubt would have toppled off the table in the fray.

All I had to do was say "Bud, DROP" and that catastrophe was completely averted. Talk about a huge sigh. So, train your dogs with the simple commands. Hopefully, you will never really need them, but you just never know.

Ace Bandages and Reader's Digest

One of the big lessons I have learned was that the tough times, the difficulties, the bumps in our road of life, serve to make us more grateful for days when things go well. It makes us appreciate the small things. For those of you who have heard my Kleenex® story, you know that I already do that somewhat. For those of you who do not know the story, I was in a foreign, third-world country with a severe sinus infection, no meds, no local currency, and no Kleenex® for three days! Now I could not be caught without a hanky at all times…

Ever since that same trip, I had also been grateful for the ease with which we had hot running water and could take a shower or bath without carrying it or heating it over a fire. Now I was appreciative of just being able to complete the act of showering without being so exhausted that the rest of my day has to be spent in bed. I was grateful for being able to wash my own hair! When I couldn't shower, I had to have help and get in an incredibly uncomfortable position to wash it. Also, when hubby washed my hair, although he did a great job, not being used to the act of washing long hair was quite a challenge for him to do a really good job. There was a silly trick to getting all the soap and conditioner out of my hair, and he struggled with that, but that was OK. He's a guy … a mostly bald guy.

I had my first, true full day yesterday, and I felt good this morning. I was thrilled. Mostly, because today was another full day ahead, and now I had confidence I could get through today and enjoy the goings on. Yesterday, I took a shower and washed my hair all by myself (gasp!), got dressed all by myself (gasp!—this was still a struggle for range of motion reasons), went shopping with a dear friend for about two to three hours, went out to lunch with her, then went out to dinner and a movie last night with hubby and some of our cousins.

I fell quite asleep before everyone left, while I was still plugged into my meds, but it was a wonderful full day.

Find a new normal.

It felt almost normal. When you go through illnesses that last longer than a week or two, especially a debilitating one, you tend to begin to feel like things will never be normal again. In many cases they never were, and you had to find a new normal. But then, when the normal returns or starts afresh there is a tremendous sense of peace about it, because you could feel yourself really getting better, or being at peace with the new normal.

So I was starting to find my new normal, finally. I hope to be off all the antibiotics in about four days. That would mean the last tube would be removed, and all I should have were my nice set of all new scars. I still had the final reconstruction and ovary removal ahead, but that seemed small potatoes after all of this. Pretty soon I would be cleared for physical therapy, and eventually I would be able to get dressed, and move without discomfort.

Discomfort. That reminds me. I have been trying to figure out how to describe what I it felt like with the expanders in. It was really strange. Most of the skin was numb. I kept bumping, scratching, and rubbing numb spots. One underarm was totally numb, which made putting on deodorant odd. Imagine trying to apply deodorant to a stranger with your eyes closed. That's kind of how it felt. I couldn't tell if I actually got enough on in the right spots or not. I spent a lot of time checking to see if I smelled or not.

There were still some spots where the nerves were deciding to either regenerate or die, and so there was a tingly, yucky feeling in a few spots as well, mostly on the underside of my upper arms. That affected dressing, because certain material was uncomfortable, but that was getting better gradually. When I first came out of my first surgery, I had nerve issues all down one arm and numbness and pain in my right hand. That was finally all better.

Now, the implants. The expanders were placed between the muscle layers in the chest. (If they are just placed under the skin without breast tissue they migrate south. Talk about saggy boobs! They would eventually migrate

so far south I would be an incredibly well-endowed male
– 'nuff said there.) So, they separate the muscle layers
from each other to create a pocket to put the implants
into. With stretching the muscles, as with any muscle, the
muscle will react. Well, when you think about it, there
was a whole lot of stretching going on. Basically, we were
stretching the muscles to the point of straining them,
allowing them to heal, and then doing it again until we
reached the right amount of space to have the permanent
implants put in. There are many sets of nerves in our
bodies; pain nerves, hot/cold nerves, pressure nerves, etc.
Most of them are on the skin, but there are some inside of
us which allow us to feel pain, such as muscle pain. So, I
could feel the pain, yet not feel the pain.

I could kind of feel the expanders, both from the inside
and out. Imagine taking a *Reader's Digest* magazine,
folding it in half and wrapping it tightly against your
chest with an ace bandage. Now, remember that a lot
of breast tissue was actually located under your arm.
So I could feel it every time I put my arm down. It was
not so much uncomfortable, as just not normal. It was
different. It felt weird, like I was walking around trying to
hold something under my arms. I suppose a part of me
subconsciously kept a tight grip, too. I did notice that I
had to consciously drop my arms often.

Lying down on my side was really different. I could
really feel the expanders then. Unlike normal body tissue
that kind of has some give to it when you lie of your side,
these didn't go anywhere. It felt a bit like I was lying on
something. For now, it still hurt a bit, but it was vastly
improved since a month ago, so I knew eventually, it

would not hurt at all. I wondered if the weird feeling would ever go away. I knew that the implants would never feel normal to touch, but I never thought about how it would feel from my perspective of them being inside my body.

Would this funky feeling of Ace bandage and *Reader's Digest* ever go away? No biggie really, just another little piece you do not think about from an outside perspective. I never would have thought to ask how that would feel. I knew at some point I would be so used to them that I wouldn't notice, but since I was not expecting to feel this way even at the start, I found it interesting.

I could now give very light hugs without pain, what a blessing! I could shower, dress, and I was gradually finding my new normal.

Life was good.

Milestones

Another milestone has been reached in my recovery: I have completed my round of Vancomycin antibiotics! YEAH! I still got to keep the PICC line in for now. The doctor was going to do blood draws in about a week to make absolutely sure I didn't have any lingering infection. That works. I still had to wrap my arm for showers, but hey, it's progress. I'll take it.

I tried to take walks around the neighborhood daily, now that the weather was nicer. Yesterday, I met two of my neighbors on the street behind me. We have woods and a gully behind our houses, and we couldn't just wave over the back fence like most backyard neighbors, so it was not surprising I had not met them in the four years I've lived here.

One of the ladies was out gardening, and we got into a lovely discussion about the challenges of gardening in our area that has a lot of clay and shade, since we were surrounded by huge trees in our neighborhood. We live in an unusual neighborhood. The trees were all older than our houses. The houses were built among the trees (how "green"). The upside was a young house with mature trees, the downside was that the trees were supposedly protected, as this area was considered to be a wildlife corridor, and we could not cut down the trees that were older than our homes unless they were dead or diseased. So, we all had to plant things that grew in full shade.

I do, however, love it in full summer when our backyard was almost a full ten degrees cooler than our front yard. We also really do not have any back neighbors that we could see, except in full winter when the leaves are gone.

Back to the subject: Meeting the neighbors. OK, so I got a great gardening lesson, and some good ideas and then proceeded on. A few doors down, a gal was out front waving good bye to someone who was driving off. I noticed a plant in her the yard that looked familiar to one in my yard, only it was much bigger, so I inquired about it.

After chitchat, I finally noticed her shirt: Race for the Cure Susan G Komen Foundation. I believe God leads us where He wants us to go. She would have only been out a moment, and had I not stopped to chat with the first lady, I would have missed this lady. For those who may not know about the Komen Foundation, they are an organization trying gain education and research for a breast cancer cure. I had stumbled across a new friend who understood my walk and was an open door for many others. Wow. I had even seen her many times in public, as it turned out, we frequented some of the same places and even knew mutual friends.

Who knows where all this may lead. It may lead to nowhere, or it may lead to all sorts of new directions. At least now I could start walking with more purpose to be a part of the race for the cure.

Perseverance

What a frustrating day. The realities of what was ahead of me were weighing heavily. Silly things like how to shave safely under my arm pits when I couldn't feel them. I was prone to rashes if I shaved too hard. I had so little range of motion in my shoulders, and even though the pain was subsiding, I could hardly put on shirts. I tried to lift a roasting pan (it was heavy, but had to weigh less than ten pounds), and I could not budge it using both hands. I have a lot of physical therapy ahead of me. This was going to be a really long year.

Top it off with my wonderful release from Vancomycin, tempered by the fact that I have come down with a cold. It's a regular head cold; a yucky, but relatively benign, infection. But, it was another infection, nonetheless. So now I was trying to control the sinuses, because I was prone to sinus infections and bronchitis, although I haven't had bronchitis in a few years. I was hoping my body was strong enough to fight off bronchitis, because

I really did not feel like a bunch of coughing, thanks though. Fortunately, my silver lining was that it did not hurt to cough any more than it used to.

I try to solace myself with the comfort that I was so fortunate not be having chemo. I would be having horrible trouble if I was. Do you realize that if my treatment was requiring chemo, I would not yet have been healthy enough to have begun it? I would have been sitting here, still fearing the cancer, and wondering when I could have treatment. I would have been wondering if I was losing my grip on cancer with all the delays in treatment. My heart goes out to those who were in that boat exactly. That is a fear I had been able to avoid, yet I did partly understand it.

I would persevere; I was just tired of having to.

So, I was going to fix myself a nice cup of tea, take another dose of my seemingly fifty million meds, crawl back into bed, and hope and pray I felt better very soon (and in better humor for the sake of my family—I'm quite grumpy right now). I would persevere; I was just tired of having to.

Tylenol and Tape

I'd finally been cleared to start physical therapy. On one hand, I was so excited because I knew I'd soon be able to regain the mobility and strength that I had lost. It has frustrated me to know just how much I had lost. I couldn't even put on a shirt over my head right now or reach for things above my head. But that would soon change. And I could hardly wait.

I knew that the therapy was going to be intense, and uncomfortable, but it was a different kind of pain than the healing of surgery. Oh, it's not going to be fun, but it's the kind of pain my grandpa said you got because you were doing something. I should be buying stock in Advil these days. I was pleased to realize that I was taking quite a bit less medication than I thought I was in regards to the strong stuff. I went in to see my regular PA (physician's assistant) to just fill him in on what I was going through, rather than him just reading my stuff from my surgeon.

That was a good thing to do, by the way. Your regular doctors receive reports from the other doctors (like surgeons), but it was all quite succinct, and details are left out. Things such as how you are handling the pain or some of your concerns, are not put in the reports. My PA was aware of my complications and how long I was in the hospital, but he was not necessarily aware of how all that affected the rest of me. My plastic surgeon knew about my implants and mastectomies. The PA knew me.

I have Epstein-Barr virus. It's a chronic condition version of mononucleosis. Yes, the dreaded kissing virus that plagued high school and college. Every once in a while, when my body was stressed, it reared its ugly head and I got to go through mono all over again (but I was not contagious anymore). It can affect the healing processes, which was why I was healing slowly, although I was healing well. My scars would take forever to fade. Where some people heal cuts in about a week, I often take two. I was sometimes prone to infections, but only when I was already in full blown mono. A small bit of damage had been done to my liver, so that was something that needed to be watched.

Our livers filter out toxins that would otherwise build up and kill us. These toxins sometimes come about as byproducts of things we eat. Tylenol® or anything with Tylenol® has to be detoxified in the liver. Since I already had scarring in my liver from the mono (it really was minor), I needed to be careful.

When the mono rears its ugly head, I feel pain in my liver. I also feel pain in my liver if there are too many toxins that it has to deal with. While I was in the hospital, I was on a lot of pain meds with Tylenol® (which, oddly enough, does nothing for me as far as pain control), I had liver pain and my meds had to be changed.

This was a good reason to remember to be your own advocate. The hospital staff, who did not know my full history, had no idea that Tylenol® might do that to me. Many of my medications had Tylenol® in them. Write stuff down if you have to for use in medical settings. My mom had so many, she eventually compiled a two-page list (or was it longer?) of procedures, diagnoses, and medications. I needed to do that now. I have all sorts of quirky sensitivities that do not affect me in regular life, but have huge impacts on me in a medical setting. Many of them were discovered recently.

> Write stuff down if you have to for use in medical settings.

You can imagine what a big deal it became when I was sensitive to adhesives on tape. I could still see the lines where the tape was from my first surgery, two months ago. They were aware this might be an issue, and used less tape, but think about it. I had tape over the incisions (Steri-strips), over the bandaging at the surgical site, over my IV line, over the drainage tubes, over the PICC line: lots of tape. The doctors just needed to be aware so they knew to watch me more carefully for reactions. My PICC line had to have tape over it for a few weeks. The skin was so tender that when they took off the tape and removed the PICC line and put a tiny Band-Aid over the hole, I got blisters from the Band-Aids. No biggie, just kind of a "you've got to be kidding me" kind of thing. So I was slathering lotion over the other areas now that I could, and all was well.

Make sure you get a good dialogue going with all your doctors, write stuff down if you must: I could never remember dosages of meds I was on. Remember that your primary doctor may not be the specialist, but he or she was going to know the most about you. Make that relationship stronger by communicating. Keep them updated, keep them in the loop. Let them know, in your words what has happened and how you are. Show them your scars. Doctors love scars. Don't let them fool you into thinking they got into medicine to help others or even for the money. It's all for the scars. Yup, that's it. It's all about the scars. They're cool.

The Good Hurt

I'm here to tell you that there is such a thing as good pain. I started physical therapy (PT) yesterday. It hurt, but felt so good at the same time. I knew I was really healing now. I was on the road to being comfortable again. I could regain my movement and put on all my normal shirts that go over the head, not button down. Eventually I would be able to lie on my side again to sleep. It was good, so good.

The stretches were not easy, nor were they fun, but I could calculate a real difference with each exercise. It was awesome! I could tell I was gaining range of motion again. Then after I stretched, I noticed that I didn't hurt so much. Yes, I had the achiness of "hey, you've been doing something," but I felt better, and did not hurt as much. I did the exercises, and I did them a lot. I did them more than the therapists said to do them, but only to my comfort level. Work, work, work. Got it done. Regain my life. Reclaim it.

I was realizing how much strength I had lost, and that too would return. Strength would be a lot harder than regaining mobility, and it would take a lot longer to get there. I knew what I was doing this summer: becoming a gym rat. By the end of the summer I'd be all buffed up walking around going "I'm going to pump (clap) you up!" OK, well, maybe I'll just be able to lift the five-pound dumbbells over my head. Either way, it was progress.

With a lot of help, I started on my garden for the year. It was not a whole lot, just cleaning up here and there, and adding a few more flowers. My son, Alex, says I need more color, so I may have to go buy some annuals to pretty up the place. I'm trying to get the garden such that something was blooming all spring, summer, and fall. Who knows? I'm not that good at gardening, but I do like to try!

I finally got my hair cut and colored again last week. I had a nice pink stripe again! Breast cancer awareness is more important than we acknowledge. Yes, we wear pink, we wear the wrist bracelets, but do we really know how many women are touched by this? I'm not going to throw numbers at you, because they would be meaningless. But I believe the reality of those numbers would be daunting.

Of course I talk a lot about breast cancer, because I had it, but we have had other cancers in our family. A cure for any cancer would lead to a cure for all cancers eventually. It's insane the amount of people who have to live with it, the fear of it, or the fear of getting it again. I get fliers all the time asking for donations to this cause or that. I had a difficult time giving to an organization simply because there was so much need everywhere, even if all of it was important. How do you choose between a cure for multiple sclerosis or cancer? Both are horrible. Both deserve to have cures found. But how do you choose?

You end up choosing based on what you have in your own life, your own experiences. Mine was cancer. My sister-in-law's was MS, which she had.

So feel free to choose. Giving to something is better than giving to nothing. Find what speaks to you, and give. Give your time, talents, and money. Give. Get involved. There is always something more to be done, and someone needing to do it. Walk for the cure, volunteer, give money, go to a fund raiser, and talk to your politicians about healthcare. Do something, because in doing nothing we all die a little quicker, and in a lot more discomfort.

Soldiering On

For those of you undergoing chemo, radiation and reconstruction (or not) for breast cancer, I salute you! I am dumbfounded by how you did it and could find a way to smile and keep going. Today was one of those days where the whole world felt like it woke up and decided I was going to have a rough day. It was one of those days where all the problems that still existed even when the cancer came along decided to remind me they were still there.

Lee was slated to start deploying pretty soon.

I didn't want to have that added stress on top of just trying to heal and take care of the boys when I still could hardly pick up any of the cats.

I was frustrated, thinking "how was I going to do all this?" Now, I know that so many of you were there to support me, and help, and I love you all for it, but I have to admit, from an independence standpoint, it was frustrating and discouraging. My range of motion was coming back slowly, but I was still not ready to try any strengthening yet.

I had to laugh today though. My poor PT. He tried something new with me today: a strength exercise. There was a stretchy band that was attached to the wall. I stood at ninety degrees, so my side was facing the wall. I had the stretchy band in the outfacing hand. Upper arm parallel to the body, lower arm ninety degrees to the body, pointing forward. All I was supposed to do was rotate my lower arm out away from my body without moving my elbow. Sounds simple? I couldn't even budge it past taut.

Sigh. OK, so not today. Maybe later.

But, we soldier on. All of us do. No one's life was perfect, or in perfect harmony. Something is always going on, some stressor of some kind, whether good or bad. It was the human condition. So be it. Sure would be nice to be calm for a while though, wouldn't it? We love to blame others, whether it be our spouse, our parent, or our government (or just the current president), when in reality, it was just life. It's not always fair, and it was not always directly someone else's fault, regardless of how it looks to us.

On a brighter note, it seems the boys got their yearbooks today. It's a sure sign of the impending end of another school year. That flew! Guess I had better figure out how to keep these ya-hoos from driving me nuts all summer. Anyone need their lawn mowed?

Progress

Progress, calculable progress, was awesome! I had almost regained all my range of motion, and my pain level was so far down that I had not taken any meds, the pain was tolerable, and it was afternoon. What a joy to not be chained to the Advil bottle. I'll probably take something now, but this was the longest I'd gone without taking anything since before surgery. I had been working hard in physical therapy, and even finally graduated from an exercise. It was amazing how wonderful it felt to graduate from an exercise that was agonizing at the start or too difficult to do. I just wanted to jump for joy. It made for good motivation to do the exercises at home simply so I could keep progressing. There was even an exercise during my last session that was introduced and it was immediately determined that I didn't need it. (I could put both hands behind my back and reach up far enough to get to the now unnecessary bra strap). I'll take it.

I was moving easier. I even had on a sweater that I pulled on over my head and got on without struggling! I would take it off slowly (I couldn't go quickly if I wanted to), but then again, husbands usually didn't complain too much about exaggerated slowness in this particular exercise. But the point being that I could get it on and off without feeling like I ripped myself open. I tell you what, I had been beginning to feel like I was never going to feel better, really better. I could now even lay, not only on my side, but my stomach. Only for short times, but I could. Joy! See, I was not a back sleeper, so it had been horrible to be stuck sleeping that way all this time.

I discovered another ally in my arsenal of tricks to help me feel better: heat packs. No one had really said I needed to be doing this or cold packs, but I decided to try it. Holy cow, I felt a lot better using heat packs! It was worth its weight in gold to have a good heat pack. I suggest getting the kind filled with rice or flaxseed that could be put in the microwave. Make sure that they have little pockets within the pack to keep the filling in place, otherwise gravity takes over and the majority of the heated filling will sit too low, and not on the top of your shoulders. Just heat packing in the evenings reduced my pain and may be helping to improve my sleep as well.

It was worth its weight in gold to have a good heat pack.

Next week would be an interesting endeavor as I would have my first fill done. This meant that this was the first time the doctor would add some fluid into the expanders. So, I got to walk in to my appointment mostly flat, and walk out with a cup size. I had no idea how much he would put in. I had no idea if it would hurt and no idea if

I would feel like I took two steps back in physical therapy or not. We would just have to wait and see. Either way, I hope to at least look more female then.

From an emotional standpoint, well, it's still a bit tough. Since I had been concentrating so much on the healing, I had not had as much time to notice the disfiguring. My scars were starting to heal enough that they became flat, rather than the jagged folded skin I was getting used to looking at. I needed to be putting Aquaphor on them, but that has been problematic, since I had to basically put stuff with the consistency of Vaseline all over my chest, and then I couldn't cover it with tape or anything. This meant I either had to (a) go topless, which hubby didn't mind, but the boys would or (b) grease up a shirt, which felt really gross. It didn't exactly make me really want to put much lotion on. Either way, the scars were continuing to heal. I kind of wish we could just leave the expanders in without replacing them, and bypass the last big surgery. I'm sure not in a hurry to go into that last surgery just yet.

We were still having unseasonably cool weather here now, as I was sitting here typing with a sweater on and was still cold. It's raining out, but at least we were not getting any bad storms. Those friends of mine in Oklahoma were not so lucky! I hope they were all safe. So much for global warming, huh?

The kids' last day of school was today. Wow, that flew by! Lee was already gone, and the boys had done a pretty good job of helping out, but thank goodness I wasn't weaker, because they really had no idea how to do stuff and what to do. No worries though! There was still plenty of work left to do for the summer.

I worked on the garden for about an hour, as I could now do light gardening work. The front garden was looking beautiful, and would be really pretty when it matured.

Come on spring. Come on summer. Gimme some sun. Gimme some warmth. This weekend was supposed to get into the nineties. I'll believe it when I see it.

First Fill

Well, I had my first filling in my reconstructive process. I admit I was dreading it. I've been a bit grumpy; tired, really. I was tired of hurting, tired of taking pain meds, and tired of feeling, well, tired. My healing was going well, mind you, but I was still combating the looming threat of a mono recurrence, and I just couldn't do anything fast. That included healing. So everything was fine, just kind of in slow motion. Consequently, I was not where I wanted to be and I was frustrated that I still hurt. Yet, I hurt so much less it's ridiculous, and I should be jumping for joy, if jumping didn't hurt.

Now, when you go in to the doctor's office, as we have all learned, and they say "this may be a bit uncomfortable," that translates to "yup, it's going to hurt." So, when the nurse says "I hope you took some pain meds," well, that didn't bode well, and I was having flashbacks to the pain of removing the first set of drainage tubes.

I took my usual dose of meds, and kind of held my breath as I went in to the office. Now, others had tried to reassure me that this really didn't hurt. After all I've been through, I was a bit skeptical.

The plastic surgeon came in, and the first thing we had to do was find the port to stick the needle into. They had a magnet in the expander port and this little hand-held detector to find the magnet. He used the detector to find the magnet in the port, and then the needle was inserted. As my doctor put it: "it says put needle here, dummy." You have to love a doc with a good sense of humor.

Well, the blasted detectors were not working right. Fortunately, the ports were not hard to palpate. It seemed strange to have my surgeon, a man who was not my husband, feeling my empty breast for a thickness that would indicate the port: Especially having this done while my husband was sitting in the room. Now, they could put in anywhere from sixty to one hundred and fifty milliliters of saline in each side at a time. So, I was thinking less was going to be less painful. I let my doc know I was not in a hurry, and we could do extra fill appointments as opposed to more pain. We decided to go off of my tolerance level. Fine.

He began to fill.

OK, I have wracked my brain for a good word to describe how that felt. Only one word came to mind: weird. There was no way to accurately describe how it felt. The good thing was, it did not hurt. Not a bit, not the needle going in, not the saline filling, nothing. However, I could feel the expander gradually unfolding. That was unreal, and as I said, weird. The closest approximation

I can think of would be to hold a large empty balloon tightly in your hand, and blow it up, while still keeping your grip tight. I'm a bit less lumpy now, but still far from smoothed out. My immediate reaction after I first saw the transitional me?

Holy crap!

Of course, I really said that out loud and right in front of my doc. I had to laugh, but he found it funny too, as did Lee. So I walked in an AAA cup, and walked out an A cup (or so). That works. But, back to the amount. Remember, I asked him to go light? That I wasn't in a hurry? I was shocked when he said he managed to easily get 150mL in each side! WHAT? But won't that, you know, hurt?

I couldn't really say that it did. Yeah! I was a bit sore, but only like I was about two weeks ago, not much of a backslide. I did have to up my meds a bit, but all that meant was that I was taking three doses of Advil® as opposed to two and back to taking codeine at night again.

And I had arm pits again. Not sure how to explain that one other than "flat" chested also included my underarm, and I didn't really have any pits. They were numb anyhow, so either way, it didn't hurt. But, now the pits were back, and I was amazed that I cared.

I teased my boys that I was going to wear a bikini top when I was done being "inflated" and drive in the jeep with the top down. Of course the boys were properly appalled. I'm so mean.

Landmarks

Today was a landmark day. I finally finished my one online class that I kept after having to drop everything else at the beginning of the semester. I could say I accomplished something tangible. I know, I know, I've sure done an awful lot already. But this was different, because I got to control this. I made this happen. I studied, I did something, and had now achieved something to show for it; a grade. Not being the type of person who has to be perfect, I got a B, and I was thrilled. I could have gone for the A, but I didn't want or need to stress myself out about the stupid final grade, when I was struggling just to finish the class.

Either way, I did it. Happy Dance.

Another landmark was that I finally was off all pain meds. I still got stiffened up in the shoulders and all, but I didn't hurt. It was wonderful. I was still far from "normal" and sleeping comfortably was still a challenge. I started sleeping with a pillow held across my chest. It gave me support when I laid on my side, and it also kept the cats from sitting right on my chest. That really helped, but it still was not what I would consider comfortable. I could finally take my shirts on and off normally with very little discomfort. My range of motion was almost all back. My strength was still poor but getting better every day, as it was finally time to push myself. I could pick up, but not carry a one gallon milk jug, and that was progress.

Something still very difficult was the realization that I was probably not going to ever be able to work with exotic cats as I had always dreamed. You need to be strong for that. You need to be able to toss around fifty pounds for that. I couldn't do that anymore. I really do not think that it is realistic to think I ever would be that strong again. And as I watched my house cats play around my feet, a part of me thought, "Who cares?" I found doing domestic cat rescue difficult, as there is such a huge over population, you have to accept that it's a losing battle. No matter what, you cannot save them all. That was an unbelievably hard concept for me, because I got so attached to each animal so quickly. Or should I clarify, not only could I not save them all, but I also could not keep them all.

For crying out loud, I couldn't even blow off the fact that my dog got into a nest of bunnies and the remaining ones were dying because of maggots. There was a part of me that just wanted to save them, but I knew I could not. I couldn't save the world, but I somehow kept trying.

I suppose that was all part of being a fighter. Fighting to do the right thing, fighting for my daughter, fighting for my marriage (although I seemed to be doing more damage than fighting right now), fighting cancer and fighting to keep the one class. I knew it was all worth it.

I just got to take a lot of interesting detours along the way that lead to some interesting places, some of which I regret, some I would not trade for the world.

Notice I said, "fighting to do the right thing"? I was referring to my marriage. Even though I was so mad at Lee, even though I was denying seeing all the wonderful things he was doing to care for me then, it did matter to me to try to do what God wanted me to do in my marriage. I prayed so much. I knew better than to pray for permission to leave the marriage, and I knew it would be wrong to pray for it to be OK to leave anyway, but that was completely how I felt. I knew in my heart I was doing something against what God wanted, but I wanted to do it anyhow. I knew how painful it would be to stay. More pain in the fight: Emotional pain in dealing with my marriage; physical pain in recovering from the cancer.

I was afraid of the pain. I knew I would to survive the fight. There was a difference. Being afraid of the fight means you doubt whether or not you would finish and win. Being afraid of the pain means you were accepting the fight, embracing it, but acknowledging that it wasn't going to be easy.

The difference, dear friends, was in trusting God to see you through to the end, but knowing it would be a challenge or whether you trust His presence in the fight. Remember that we do not know God's will for us. Even if we did, who was to say we would understand it anyhow? We need to put our faith in His wisdom, plan, and purpose, and walk in confidently like David into our battle with Goliath. David did know he would win, but he didn't know if he would get hurt. He went anyway. So should we.

Second Fill

I had my second fill the other day. Not much different than the first. I'm rounder, less bumpy, and definitely a lot closer to my previous size. Everyone is too polite to tell me if I look about the same or not. Then again, I had been warned that the expanders were not going to look quite right, and to just suck it up and not worry, because the permanent implants look a ton better, whatever that means.

I did not need pain meds, just some Advil. I was still achy, and my skin was really tight, but that was to be expected. I got in another one hundred milliliters in one side and about one hundred twenty milliliters in the other side. Clothes were fitting better as far as shirts, so that was a plus. I had one bad night's sleep afterward, but by the next night I was fine. So improvement was still steady.

I do feel exhausted. I over-did it yesterday to test my endurance limits. PT was yesterday, then a doctor's appointment with Alex, both in the morning. After that we went to the "Bodies" exhibit, you know, the one where the bodies are actually preserved bodies. The exhibit was educational and fascinating! Seeing it in a book was nothing like seeing it for real and really getting to understand how it all goes together. They did a fabulous job of being respectful in the exhibit, and it was truly interesting to learn as much as we did. Even the boys loved it. Then some dear friends came over for dinner. They were the one couple who we had known, and lived close to for the better part of seventeen years. We had a great night just hanging out and chatting.

Today, I was paying for it! I was so tired I just wanted to go back to bed, but I couldn't. My mind was too busy, and I was spending a good amount of time praying. Alex and I had another doctor's appointment. Now, as I mentioned, we had two cancers in my family that seemed to plague us, breast cancer and melanoma. So lumps and questionable moles always make us very nervous.

Alex, who was fourteen, had a questionable mole. I was sure it was all good, I had faith, but it did elicit some anxiety anyhow, just to go through the process of removing the mole and then awaiting the results. It does not bother me as much when it's me, but it does when it's my son. Like I said, I had faith that it would all be fine. I'm more concerned about him feeling confident in regard to the fact that he doesn't like needles. This would be interesting. He had had quite strong reactions before to needles. Pray for peace, strength, and getting through this. After all, no matter what, we were a family of stubbornly strong survivors.

Perky or Flat Tires?

I ended up not finishing this note yesterday simply because I didn't know where to end. The mole removal was blessedly uneventful, and Alex now has five little stitches where the mole was. He was relieved that I was not telling him tales when I said it would not hurt. He felt well enough to have a sleep over with a friend last night. That works for me.

I noticed that with this latest fill, my skin was very tight, and shiny. I'm starting to put lotion on at night to help with that, but I hate the goopy feeling and the gooiness it leaves on my shirts. I knew my doctor wanted me in there each week, but I was just not in that much of a hurry. This way, also, I could stretch more between visits, making it easier to put more in per fill. Seemed to me, I could then have fewer appointments.

I still had a very bizarre sensation each time I did anything that flexed the pectoral muscle. The feeling was similar to a big twitch, where the muscle was probably contracting around the expanders and filling in any "gaps." At least, that was my guess. I got that impression by seeing it in the mirror. OK, imagine standing in front of the mirror doing the typical boy checking his pecs in the mirror scenario. Yes, you can laugh here. I have these folds, or gaps, or indents; not sure how to describe them. If I had a larger build, I might liken it to a fat roll on the side of my breast. I was not sure if these would go away with subsequent fillings, or if this was going to be the norm. I found that the area the tubes sat in were still, well, there. I could feel the area as if there was still a residual tract. At least they were not tender anymore. I did wonder if they actually were the tops of the implants.

So, the question of the hour these days was silicone or saline. It seemed obvious to me that my doctor preferred silicone. He said the shape and feel was more normal. I assume his wife has silicone (KIDDING! Sort of.). The biggest difference was if they rupture. If the saline ruptures, it drains, the body absorbs it, and you got the "flat tire" look. Fixing it required surgery, which was fairly simple, as they take the old one out and replace it. With the silicone, ruptures would ooze out, but stay together, and your shape changed. It also required surgery to fix, which was more in depth as they had to clean out the area that oozed before putting in a new implant. Neither one would cause infections if they ruptured (so I was told), and you could tell they ruptured by the look of them rather than getting ill.

I still need to research the rates at which the implants "decay" and rupture. If there was a significant difference between the two, that needed to be thrown into the mix. If saline was easier to replace, but needed to be replaced approximately every ten to fifteen years, as opposed to silicone, which needed replacing about every twenty to twenty-five years, I might decide the more involved surgery was better than more surgeries within the remainder of my lifetime.

Now, when I was old and grey (but still perky), and the implants failed, could they just be left in? Probably not the silicone, but what about the saline? After all, old ladies were supposed to have their boobs heading south to their knees. Could I get the other type if I did have to have them replaced? (The answer is yes.) Always more questions.

Stretch Marks
and Sadness

Today was a tough day. I found out a friend of mine, a dear elderly lady who has my utmost respect and love, was dying of cancer. Not a day goes by that I forget that not everyone beats back this disease. My battle was easily won this time, and it wasn't easy. I knew that there were some who would not live to see another healthy, pain-free day. And it sucks. And it hurts. And it makes me feel guilty, even though I shouldn't feel guilty. This was a lady I never took the time I should have to glean so many wonderful truths of life that I knew she had. Her husband was a wonderful, and decorated, retired Air Force General. They both were the epitome of loving, faithful Christians, who raised equally wonderful children. She was one of those people that seemed to have it all figured out. She was never in doubt, always trusted God, and was always happy, unless she was crying with you over the unfairness of the world. She could tell the heart of a person, and would tell you she was praying for you when you needed it most.

She has been kind of like the matriarch of our church in a way. She would be so dearly missed. She was terribly missed merely on days she was not in church. This was hard on the whole church and community.

I couldn't sleep. At least not well. I couldn't get comfortable. It's not so much that it hurt as much as it felt like I had to sleep on rocks. If this was what saline feels like, it might just be worth it to get silicone after all. Then maybe I could get some sleep.

I also had some new friends I had picked up along the way. I needed to call them friends and accept their walk with me, because they were unwelcome but not going anywhere, so I just had to suck it up: Stretch marks. Not a surprise at all, but not really what you want either. Now my breasts were scarred, warped, and tender in some spots and numb in others, swollen and had stretch marks all over them. Sigh. At least I look OK in clothes, or would in a few weeks.

On the bright side, all the stretch marks on my top now matched the stretch marks on my bottom (thighs specifically). Balance was the key, right? Since I was naturally kind of pear shaped, I wonder how I'd look if the top matched the bottom. I'd probably fall over all the time. Gee, they really look more like lightning than anything. Why couldn't we call them "lightning strikes"? Sounds more, I don't know, exciting? "I have lightning strikes," versus "I have stretch marks." Maybe that was worth consideration.

Lee deployed, and as usual the gremlins have infested within the forty-eight hour time frame. The dishwasher is broken. We need a new one. Nice. I would have asked what else would go wrong, but I was scared to ask.

Finding New Dreams

I was looking at a new site that I really liked on Facebook called, "Beyond the Boobie Trap." It was not so much about breast cancer as about finding your new normal, after all was said and done. Boy, was that a good point. I had the opportunity to talk with site's creator, and it was a fun, upbeat conversation. We were similar ages with several other surprising similarities. She really hit the nail on the head when she said that when you were in treatment, you had a team. Your oncologists (the cancer doctors), your regular doctors, radiologists, infusion teams for chemo, physical therapists, plastic surgeons, therapists, etc. Then, when it was all over, and you were healing, and all was said and done, all those sources were suddenly gone. Now, there was a part of you that was thrilled and never wanted to see any of them again (simply because that would mean you were sick again). But then what? Your old life, your old normal, was gone. You were you, but not you. You had to get used to the scars, the new aches and pains, swollen body parts due to having lymph nodes removed. Clothes didn't fit right; nothing felt right. And who was this person looking back at you in the mirror? The only thing the same was the eye color, and even your eyes had lost that old gleam.

Finding the new normal was a very difficult task. For me, all the things I had planned for the next five years went out the window the day I got diagnosed. All of it, gone. So, now what? What do I do when I have to start from scratch? What do I do when everything has turned to mush? Well, the very first thing I did was put pink stripes in my hair. I'm not a tattoo person (does anyone really look good at eighty-years old with a tattoo?), but hair grows. Since I blessedly missed chemo, and got to keep the hair, I had pink stripes. Not a ton, I do not look like a zebra, but I do have two stripes. I like them, and several others that I know had followed suit. Neat.

Buying clothes was interesting. Shirt sleeves were still very uncomfortable, and that affected how I dressed. So I guess, on the bright side, I got to reinvent my style: New textures, fits, and fashions.

I went to Goodwill a fair amount since I couldn't afford a totally new wardrobe immediately; besides, I was still trying to figure out what I like and could wear. I didn't want to spend a mint on nice new clothes that I could not wear. That had been happening quite a bit as things shrank just that little bit in the wash. Ahem. No, of course I didn't actually gain weight. It's the wash, I tell you. I have to admit, it's a fair reason to go clothes shopping with a friend or two.

And then we would have to have to have the cup of coffee afterward, of course. Getting together with my friends was paramount. I had been so blessed by the number of friends that I had who were there for me. Coffee wasn't just coffee. To me, it was a symbol of the friendships I helped create. I didn't get to see everyone I wanted to, but I sure got to see a lot of them every once in a while. We always had coffee when we got together, as well as at Bible study. I hadn't been able to go in ages, and I missed that. My energy levels were not up to snuff yet, and evenings I really dragged starting at 1900. That was usually when Bible study started. But I had coffee in the mornings with some of them, and we talked about our illnesses, families, faith, friendships, all the ills of the world, and all the blessings in it as well. Some of those relationships really strengthened. I would not say any of them had really faltered, but I kind of knew where I stood before all this happened anyhow.

The military spirit in me was chomping at the bit to move again. After all, we've been in the same house for four years: come on! But then I sit on my back porch, overlooking the woods behind me, and listening to the peacefulness inside it, and I think about all my relationships here. OK, I'll stay put a bit longer. But I do miss my family in California, and I miss nice weather year around there.

I love being out in the open, away from the stresses of population, and getting back to some semblance of nature. There was amazing healing in nature and amazing healing in the simplicity of camping. With that being said, my forest in my own backyard was calling me. Enjoy your day.

Tossing Cats

Last night, it was raining so much and so hard that there were flood warnings all over. I couldn't sleep without heavy meds because I couldn't get comfortable. If I didn't sleep, I was at risk for waking the sleeping giant of my Epstein-Barr virus (chronic mono), and then the fun would really start.

The sleep issue was simply that no position was comfortable to go to sleep in. I used to be a side or stomach sleeper. Those days were gone for now. I was not a back sleeper. I still used about six pillows on the bed to help prop me into a comfortable position at all hours of the night. Nothing worked for long. I could not count the number of times I woke up during the night.

Then of course, comes the dreaded can't go back to sleep, and your mind turns on, and you start thinking about all the stress happening, and then you really wake up. Then you look at the clock, it's only 0345. Joy. Now you struggle to get back to sleep, but by then you are awake enough to go to the bathroom. In my house, that was the cue for the cats to insist on being fed. So now, it's the middle of the night, and although my bladder is now empty, the cats are swarming, rubbing my legs, tripping me as I try to navigate back to bed in the dark; very difficult to do when I had dark colored cats. Then they yowl at me as I stumble back towards the bed and mumble that it is not time for breakfast, and they would have to deal.

Then the fun would really start: getting comfortable again. First: getting back into bed. That consisted of tossing and or lying on the cats that were previously under foot, but were now on the bed. This was ongoing, as they tend to yo-yo right back up onto the bed whenever they were displaced. Someday, I expect to hear a "crunch" as I fall into bed when one of them refuses to move.

Second: finding a comfy position. Yeah, good luck with that. As soon as I found something half-way comfortable, the cats would descend once again, trying to claim a comfy spot of their own, which was usually on top of me and therefore, not comfy for me. Of course, this begs the simple question of why not toss the cats from the room, right? Wrong. When they are denied full access to the bedroom they sit and scream a chorus of dissatisfaction and try woefully to open the door by banging, scratching and pawing under the door, and knocking stuff over in the hallway. During the day, when I was not tired, it was hilarious to listen to the lengths they would go. However, in the middle of the night, it was disruptive to sleep.

Well, here I should have a third, by English writing protocol, but darned if I could remember a number three. My head was a bit fuzzy from lack of sleep. Did I mention that I was not sleeping well? So, we we'll skip number three.

My memory was shot since surgery number one, and I was convinced it had something to do with the meds they used on me. Not that I was blaming the doctors for anything going wrong, just trying to figure it out. Chemo totally screws with your brain, and a lot of people get what they call "chemo brain." I would like to say that was what was happening, except that I'm not on chemo. Could we call it "cancer brain" and go with that? Whatever. I just wanted to crawl back into bed and get a good night's sleep. It looked like that was not going to be possible for a long time.

Sigh.

I'll be calling my doc today to discuss sleep aids. The last thing I needed was to fight the mono too, because it screws with the body's healing processes, and having the next surgery while the mono was active was a recipe for a long recovery. Sleep was a pretty simple thing to do to keep the mono at bay, so I would get some sleep. Somehow.

Sleeping on Rocks

I was looking at the calendar. It's the beginning of July. Six months ago, my future looked unbelievably different than it does now, and admittedly, I do too (at least sans clothing…). I was realizing that it had been about six months since my last mammogram. You know, the one that found my cancer. I had been having mammograms every six months, so I actually out of habit, thought "I better get another mammogram!" Then, of course, the absurdity of the comment hit me, and I had to laugh. When I was done laughing, my next thought was "Was I still supposed to get mammograms?"

Let's think about this for a moment, really. OK, I do not have mammaries anymore, so it would stand to reason that I would not need another mammogram. Ever. However, experiences in life had taught me otherwise. My mom had a mastectomy, and yet she got cancer again in the same breast, as a bit of tissue had been left behind. So, I ask again, do I need one? I knew the technique for the surgeries had been improved since hers, but had the necessity for continuing to look for the dreaded enemy, that was my Goliath, gone away? Has this Goliath been unequivocally vanquished? Do I still need to be watching?

Not sure. Still it does not scare me. I would be ever watchful, and I would beat it back as many times as it tried to defeat me. It was something I was raised to do; to fight. To meet me, you would think I was this little petite, social gal with nutty sense of humor, a bit meek, with a hint of insanity and fragility. Well, in truth I was one heck of a fighter, but that does not come out except when I really think it needs to. When I finally get riled up, it's time to duck and cover. Cancer would bring that out in me in a heartbeat, along with mistreating those I cared about. The thing that made me the angriest was when I could do nothing.   For some of us with cancer, that was exactly what we feel like. Helpless. How do you fight against your own body, which seems to be self-destructing? Faith, a sense of humor, and will to live: that was how you fought. But it was still easier said than done.

I decided that, after my third fill, I was pretty close to the size I was before surgery. How could I tell? Somehow just looking didn't do it anymore. I was not off balance. I could stand up from a chair without a 1-2-3-HOIST! Clothes seemed to fit normally or closer to normal than they had been. It was kind of nice. So did that mean after the next one I would be falling forward? If I fell, would I bounce back up, or would I pop the balloons? Guess I would find out.

I know, don't get them too big. I didn't want back problems and all. But I had to admit, I had never had problems with guys not listening to what I was saying because their eyes were further south. Come to think of it, they didn't seem to find much in what I was saying, either. Perhaps it would be nice to keep their attention, even if they were not listening to what I was saying, but because of what was jutting out in front of me.

That was the fun of expanders, I could try them out larger, but have smaller ones put in. So, should I have a bit of fun, and find out what it was like to get that kind of attention? I always felt as if I had to prove I had a brain, because I never seemed to keep much attention otherwise. With the obvious exception of my husband, of course, and I had always told him his glasses prescription must be off.

Bed time was gradually becoming less dreaded as the expanders were gradually feeling less and less like rocks in my chest. It was becoming easier to find a more comfortable position to sleep in. This was one of the ways in which I was discovering my new normal. My sleep was changing. I found it harder to fall asleep and stay asleep, and I was waking up earlier than I wanted but taking longer to actually get out of bed.

When I was in high school, our running coach asked us to take our pulse when we woke up, before climbing out of bed. I couldn't do it, because the minute my alarm went off, I was on my feet. Strange, I know. I discovered there were few others like me in this way. I was a total morning person. So much so that we used to have a joke about me: Sarah didn't need to get drunk, just keep her up after 2230, you'll get the same effect! Having never been drunk, nor woken up in strange places, I had to take their word for it, but I do become rather loopy (OK, loopier than usual), after that hour. So taking longer to fall asleep (many times now well after 0100), and then hopping right out of bed in the morning was now a bit unusual for me. Some might consider it an improvement, except that I was still about worthless after 2000. I stay in some drowsy twilight sleep until real sleep takes me.

I do not know if this was normal for all cancer patients, but it was for me. I really do feel like the odd duck out since I was able to avoid chemo and radiation. It was like I was part of the club, yet not part of the club. I was free to talk about the body changes of reconstruction, but felt I had no right to talk about how hard things were, when what I had to go through was "easy."

> I was part of the club, yet not part of the club.

Then I would remember, the only reason I had it "easy" was because my mom did not have it easy, and I had learned from her how to fight this even before I got it. I was proactive. I was looking for it. I knew it was coming, and I knew I would beat it. I did.

I was prepared and not afraid. I was a trained soldier on point defending my station from the potential of a threat that loomed. It reminded me of how the guards may have felt in South Korea at the DMZ, where I got to visit once. The threat loomed, but it was not "there" every day, You could never drop your guard or there it would be, sneaking past the wires and under the fence. So you watched, you anticipated, but you did not live in constant fear. Merely constant awareness, and preparedness.

Soldier on…

Bucket List Dreams

The other day, one of my boys made the comment that I was "done" with my cancer. No, I'm not. I don't say that flippantly, nor do I say that meaning I had more surgery ahead (although I did). To me, this was the beginning. Part of having cancer was the awareness of the possibility of recurrence. This does not scare me, just like getting cancer in the first place did not scare me. Why? Most would say it was because I had always been a bit odd. Others might think I'm a pessimist. Actually, I am a realist in this area. That didn't mean I was going to lie down and let it happen, any more than I did in the first place. I would be proactive. I would keep my ears open about all the things to watch for with the different cancers. I would try to remember sunscreen if I was doing more than just watering the lawn. I would get check-ups. I would get all the necessary testing done. I would not let my doctors tell me it was nothing if I was not satisfied it was nothing. I would take care of myself.

Doctors can feel lumps all they want, but they cannot definitively say it is something or nothing without a biopsy. You cannot tell by touch alone. As any woman will tell you, those individual mammary glands get rock hard sometimes when they are blocked or when we're in the middle of our cycles. That didn't mean there was cancer. Also, finding those painful lumps didn't mean it was nothing either. Every once in a while, I have an inflamed lymph node under my arm. It really hurts. It is harmless most of the time, but I watch them, and if they persist for more than three days I'm in the doctor's office going over what course of action we are taking. Sometimes it was a wait and see, other times it meant getting a better look at things.

If you are scared, don't let the doctors tell you it's just a fatty tumor (which was a diagnosis), if they had not done anything to test this. What would you rather have? A biopsy to confirm that you were fine, or would you rather take his word and have it be cancer that goes undiagnosed? Take your pick. I'll have the mildly unpleasant biopsy, thanks. A dear friend passed away because the cancer spread before they found it. What had she been told? That it was just a cramp in her leg.

I would not sit and wait and worry for the recurrences that may come my way. I would go on living how I always had to the best of my ability. I would do my best to keep my soldiers on watch for Goliath, but I would not stress over it. That would detract from my life now.

I had not done anything truly outrageous since my diagnosis. Many cancer veterans do. Many of us had a smack of our own mortality like a cold, wet, slimy fish upside the head, and decide to immediately fulfill one of our life long dreams. Kind of like the bucket list.

I bring this up because yesterday, I saw my dream car for sale. The bucket list part of me was jumping up and down going "BUY IT! BUY IT! BUY IT!" Yet the rational "I'm not giving up so easily" side of me was going "You really don't need it, it's not reasonable financially, nor for a family of four. Not now."

So, what was the car? It was an unbelievably sexy 1979 black T-top Chevy Corvette. It looked to be in great shape and was only $7000. Pardon me, while I clean up the drool on the floor. I think that if the boys had been older I would have been the brand new owner of a gorgeous Corvette. You have got to get a personalized plate for a car like that. Hmm ... let's see:

- FITE PNK
- PINK RBN
- BKT LIST
- MY DREAM
- NVRGVUP
- LIVSTRNG
- ISRVIVD
- ME1CNCR0 (OK, too long, but I love the idea)
- I LIVE

And then I had to add one that was just plain me: BLK CAT.

So, what's your vote?

I Love a Reason to Laugh

When a woman has mastectomies, how she feels about her body changes. We lose not only part of our femininity, and a function of being female (breastfeeding), but the whole concept of breasts being a sexual organ goes away. Suddenly, the breasts are about as sexual as our elbows. Do we hide our elbows from everyone for modesty sake? No. Why? Because there is nothing sexual about an elbow, and frankly, if you think there is, you need help. We tend to get this attitude about our breasts after mastectomies, even if we have reconstruction. They don't feel the same, they don't ever look the same, and well, they're just different.

Now, that being said, it would make sense that should a woman with mastectomy scars be seen topless, it is not as big of a deal to us as when we had the original pair, as far as the modesty factor. Before surgery, it was an absolute travesty to be seen by a stranger during a wardrobe malfunction. After surgery, it becomes "Hey, wait a minute! The other side looks weird, too!" It's tempting to want to whip up my shirt around my friends and ask "So, was this size good for me, or do I still need to go bigger?" And, bless their hearts, I had done just that to some of my friends who understand me well enough.

Is it OK to laugh? Of course.

I love a reason to laugh. That being said, I am really not a prankster (which can be totally confirmed by my best friend of thirty-five years, who is a prankster). I do, however, love doing things that tend to shock other people into wondering about my sanity. I'm rarely over the top with things, thus the two pink stripes in my hair versus a totally pink head.

A good reason to laugh? Take the best T-shirt I ever saw, for example. I was standing in line in the grocery store and the guy in front of me was wearing a shirt that said "Chicks dig pale, scrawny, bald guys." He fit the description exactly! What was even funnier was watching everyone around him, painfully aware of what the shirt said, and how he fit that description. Their looks were mingled with the attitude of "Is it OK to laugh?" That was the funniest part. Did I laugh? No, and I admit that I regret it to this day. We would have all been rolling, and I'm sure the T-shirt guy would have been right there with us. I still laugh when I remember that shirt, especially since it describes my hubby as well.

So, yes, it's OK to laugh. We need to laugh. For many of us, when we stop laughing, we start crying. We have too much life left to live to spend it crying, so help us get a laugh.

Close and Far

Well, I was getting closer and closer to my "normal" size, or at least to the size that would become my new normal. I had to admit, this last fill hurt. None of the other ones hurt like that. I've been pondering it for a while as to why this one was different, and may have figured it out, but I need to ask my doctor. I thought we were stretching scars on the inside. Stretching scar tissue was much harder, and more uncomfortable than stretching regular tissues. The scar tissues were very fibrous, strong, and stiff. It's like the difference between stretching a bungee cord, and stretching a rope. To stretch the rope you have to break down some of the fibers. So that would account for the pain and discomfort.

OK, look, it hurts. I needed a few Advil® to get through my day, but nothing major. I was not writhing while in agony or anything dramatic. I was not sure how the next fill would be, but time would tell. According to my doctor I only had a few left anyhow.

The time for mentally preparing for the next surgery was just around the corner, maybe two to three months away. I would admit that I was not ready. I was not looking forward to it. Yes, I wanted to get this over with and get on with my life, I just wish it didn't involve yet another surgery. Oh well. It's all part of the game. I realize that some women chose not to do reconstruction, and if I had done that, I would be well on my way to finding my new normal, and not still in the process, because I would have had the ovaries yanked by now. But we all chose our own paths for our own reasons, and that was OK. There were consequences for each of those choices. Then, there was the fact that it was the middle of July. So? Well, as any stay-at-home parents will tell you, from the end of July until school starts, the kids are bored, unhappy, fighting, cranky, and always expecting someone else to entertain them, even when they are teenagers. For my own sanity I was going to have to get creative. I started thinking, if they were so bored, they could help me clean the house and we could do some chores. I liked that. There was nothing like work to get the kids to prefer to find their own ways to entertain themselves. As far as the fighting, well, any ideas?

Oh, I remembered the other thing I wanted to touch on: touch. As I had mentioned, I had a lot of numbness. On the breasts themselves I could not feel touch, nor pressure, but could still feel pain. This was tough to explain clearly, but I'll try. I could not feel if something was hot or cold. I could not feel if something was soft, or silky. I could not feel if something was poking me, but I would still feel pain if I hurt myself. So, let's put this together a bit. I was constantly banging these new boobs into doors, because I could not perceive how close I was to them. But yet I would have momentary pain after I had bumped them. I had leaned in close to tell someone something, and discovered that I was pressing up against them, because I couldn't tell I was that close. Now I had to remember to be careful if I wanted to whisper into someone's ear.

I started mentioning this so that I could beg your pardon for winging these new things around and whapping you with them. I was simply not aware. Kind of like how women were when carrying a large purse though a crowded room. Constantly bumping people and saying excuse me. That was how I felt with the new but temporary boobs. I had a changing dynamic of where my personal-space bubble was, and was trying to adjust. First, my space bubble shrank, and now it was growing. This was hard to get used to so fast. I suppose it's similar to the awkwardness my boys felt when they got these massive growth spurts, where they woke up and looked as if they spent the night on the rack. They were gangly, with longer arms, legs, bigger hands and feet that suddenly didn't catch the ball like they used to.

My balance was a bit off, and I couldn't tell how close I actually was to what was in front of me or to the side when I had to suddenly turn a corner. Sigh. I would adjust, but in the meantime, when I go to whisper something in your ear, and totally rub up against you, forgive me. I was not hitting on you, nor was I trying to get your attention. I merely was not aware of where I was. Sorry.

I Love Me

I had this calendar that I bought around Christmastime when I was in a particularly dour mood. It's a stupid calendar. A really stupid calendar. It's an "I love me" kind of thing. It's a daily calendar with places to mark your level of self-love, or self-involvement. It has your mantra for the day, a rank of how beautiful you look that day, and a (usually) narcissistic quote from someone along the lines of Marilyn Monroe or Imelda Marcos. It's just something that gives me a chuckle, especially to think that there were actually people out there who had this calendar and filled it out religiously (I know you exist, don't deny it!).

Every once in a while, a quote would appear that actually had some real validity, especially for me. There was one of those just the other day from Sir Arthur Conan Doyle. Although I could not completely agree with the first part of the statement, I thought the last part of the statement had more truth to it than I ever gave myself credit for. I know many of us are in the same boat:

"I could not agree with those who rank modesty among the virtues ... To underestimate one's self was as much a departure from the truth as to exaggerate one's own powers." – Sir Arthur Conan Doyle

I still think modesty is a virtue. However, he was totally right in that it was not any better to diminish one's self-worth any more than it was right to embellish it. It's something I really never thought of. I always worried that I was arrogant when I was confident, and that was not something to be proud of, but in doing that I had over the years neglected to give myself credit for the things that I did well. That reality hit home terribly when I was in the veterinary technician program. We were in the surgery portion of things, and that phase has a ton of work to do outside of class. Now, I was not available for as long as the others after classes because of my own children, so I would come in early to work on stuff. No one else from my class was ever in that early. The only ones there were those whose job it was to clean the cages that week. Classes started at 0800. I was in by 0615 each day. Surgery was Thursday. During those mornings I was prepping the surgical suite by making sure everything was properly stocked, all the machines had all the proper plugs, and were located in the proper places. I was always cleaning up after everyone else and I was the only one who ran the autoclave, the machine that sterilizes the surgical instruments. I did that. I never said anything to anyone because I figured that my efforts were obvious and would be noticed. Surgery day came, and I was exhausted afterward. By then I had put in probably about fourteen to sixteen hours' worth of work in the surgery room. So when it came time for the "group" cleaning after surgery, I didn't do too much because I had already done the lion's share, and I was ready to drop from exhaustion.

Well, guess what? I got docked major points for not being a team player. None of my teammates could run the autoclave, I was doing it in my sleep and could tell you where everything in the surgical suite was located, but I was tagged a slacker. All that because no one knew it was me doing all the work. They just took it for granted that it was getting done, and I didn't speak up because I didn't want to seem like I was bragging. Lesson learned there. Not a mistake I would make again.

I did still have problems trying to balance confidence with arrogance though. I had a tendency to unintentionally speak as if I knew a subject well, when often I didn't. It's a product of debate training. It's a good thing many times, but a really bad thing because I'm sure I come off as arrogant, and a know it all. A Hermione Granger.

> There was nothing arrogant about saying I beat cancer.

So, what does that have to do with the cancer? I find myself saying "yes, I beat cancer, no biggie." Who was I kidding? I kept saying "well, my battle has been easy." And then I look in the mirror. There was nothing arrogant about saying I beat cancer. There was nothing to be ashamed of in having these huge scars across my chest.

Would a soldier be ashamed of his bullet scars? Of course not. Scars were something to be proud of and shown to every available cutie, and the good ones even got bragging rights among the other soldiers. They went to war, they paid a price, they lived, they did their jobs, and they made it home. They were heroes. OK, let me say here that any good soldier would never tell you he or she was a hero. They would say the ones who didn't come home were heroes or that someone else was a hero, not them. But that does not diminish their sacrifice!

So tell me, why should we breast cancer colleagues consider ourselves any less heroic? We are all heroes. We were put into this horrible situation without a choice. Our enemy was totally unseen; it was within our own bodies. We could not carry any means of protecting ourselves from this enemy. Any treatment would do as much, if not more, damage than the cancer itself.

I admit that I got very upset with my husband at one point. He was stationed in Iraq at the time of my diagnosis. Not a good place for him to be in the first place, and not a good place for me when he was there, and I had to get the cancer diagnosis without him home. (Again, yes, I was OK, but what if this news had been devastating? How many other wives had been in my boat?) He made some comment about how bad it was to be in a combat zone. It ticked me off. Why? Because the comment was made without the least thought about the fact that he could leave the combat zone, come home, and he was safe. When could I say I had left the combat zone?

Now, I was not belittling war zones and the horror of them. I was merely pointing out that wars were places you could get away from. Physically. There were places that you could be that were not at war. Thanks to our soldiers, I live in such a place. When the cancer was in your body, your body becomes the battle zone and you cannot escape, not even for a vacation.

Whoever has faced cancer, you are soldiers and survivors of your own personal war. Never forget that, and never neglect the fact that you were stronger than you believed. Wear those scars with pride, not shame. Those scars are a sign that you fought and survived. They are your own badges of honor. Be proud of yourselves and all you have accomplished. It may not feel like it in the midst of treatment, but one day the treatment will be over, and you will be different, but stronger and still beautiful. Be proud of that. You are a veteran.

Surgery and Peri-menopause

Stress relief was so important. It will make or break you when you have cancer. Attitude is everything. But even the best of us have bad days. Days when we feel like the bear got us. It was a gorgeous day outside, hot (which I love), not terribly humid or buggy, with a slight breeze. But I realized I felt the anxiety of my next surgery creeping up on me. I had the power to schedule when it would be next. I had the power to set the date. After that, I only needed to heal and move on. No more fills, no more surgeries ahead (that were planned anyway). I would be "done." But I was just not looking forward to having more IV's, more pain meds, more physical therapy, more needing to be taken care of. I wanted to be done with that now. I felt like a toddler, with drooping eyes, and a cranky disposition, stamping my feet and screaming "I don't need a nap!"

I knew I had to do this.

I had probably two to three months to get this done. I was surprised that when I was first diagnosed my response was "how fast can you get me into surgery?" By the time I was ready for the expander replacement, it

206 WHERE'D I PUT MY BOOBS?

had now become "do we have to do it that soon?" What a change. Weird, really. I guess it was kind of the unknown versus the known. Women, or anyone for that matter, who had been through this before knew what was ahead would rather not go through it again. Was the second time around worse than the first because you knew what was coming? That certainly explains the extreme anxiety some people feel about recurrences.

I had to also admit that I wondered if the breasts' removal triggered some perimenopause. I had mood swings, and I seemed to be having hot flashes (not sure about those because since I was always cold, it felt good...), my cycle was off, and I felt like I was going to pull a Linda Blair and find my head spinning out of control at times. If this was an inkling of menopause, I felt so sorry for my boys. Hubby would no doubt be deployed, so I would not need to feel sorry for him.

Still steadfastly refusing to see all that Lee had done for me, I remained mad. I was still done. By this point, I was beginning to look for a new place to live. I was contemplating the idea of what would become of my business, and trying to figure out what I would need to survive, and how it all might look. I was also stressing about what the future might hold for me in the sense that I am not one who likes to be alone. I did not want to get into a new relationship, but I wanted to be reassured I was beautiful and attractive. Lee never faltered in letting me know he thought I was still beautiful, but I blindly, stupidly, didn't care. I still wanted to leave him and "find someone who cared about me." It's amazing how blind one could be in one's anger.

Take Care

As I sit here, preparing for my day, trying to sip my coffee, make my eyes focus and fingers function, I was grossed out by seeing yet another pair of used rubber bands from my son Fred's braces sitting inches from the keyboard (and my coffee).

Yum. My tummy was feeling a bit upset anyhow, and this wasn't helping. The good news of that was those days should be over soon. His teeth had finally aligned, and he had an appointment tomorrow where, hopefully they would be telling us when he got his braces off. Ideally, if he would have followed the orthodontist's directions properly, he would have gotten them off a year ago like his brother. But, apparently he liked having braces enough that we decided he was planning on getting married in them several years from now and was just biding his time until then. I guess he finally figured out that it wasn't so cool to have them on forever after all, because he started doing a great job of remembering to put on the bands, and now we hoped to hear good news tomorrow. Next, he would have retainers to contend with, and remember to wear, and not throw away. One hurdle at a time, Mom.

His situation with his braces reminded me of how important it is to take care of ourselves, not just during times of illness, but at all times. Caring for ourselves could help prevent illness. There is so much involved in life, and we tend to neglect ourselves in lieu of all of life's other responsibilities. By the way, do I still classify myself as ill? The cancer was gone, but the treatments, i.e. surgeries, were not over quite yet.

Take our diets for example. Nothing makes people roll their eyes more than when people talk about eating what is good for them, and then reach for their donuts and lattes. I was not exempt. My biggest comfort food and weakness was McDonald®'s fries and nuggets. To me, those tastes with a chaser of Dr. Pepper® were heaven. However, did you know that a number eleven off of that menu I just ordered from comes with (get this!) a whole week's worth of fat (and that was the bad fat, not the good fat), and way more than our recommended daily dose of sodium!   One week's worth of fat in one sitting, and I wasn't even competing on the *Man vs. Food* show either. When I really sit with that, it's just plain gross.

Does it stop me? Of course not, but it makes me aware that I need to do better than that. On a good day of self-control, I could order the Happy Meal® version, and get only two days' worth of fat, instead of a whole week's worth and still get the emotional satisfaction of my comfort food. I don't do that as often as I should.

One of the biggest things I took away from my nutrition class was to remember that the closer the meal was to the source of the food, the healthier it was. For example, homemade apple pie is healthier than a store bought apple pie because you not only knew what went into it, but also there were no preservatives, nor any chemicals made in any labs. That was not to say that apple pie was a healthier choice than say, a no sugar/low sugar apple crisp, but either way, the point was, homemade was better. Just eating a fresh apple was healthier still.

OK, now I would have people argue that they work too much and didn't have the time to cook. Well, first off, fresh fruits and veggies and salads require almost as little time to fix as microwaving that TV dinner. Not every meal has to be fancy to be healthy, nor does it have to take long to fix, either. One of the best dinners I make is a roast chicken with mashed potatoes, fresh veggies/salad, and fresh fruit. The actual time it takes me in the kitchen is just over 30 minutes. Cooking time is about two hours, and if that is a problem, that is what crock pots are for! Point being, working was no excuse for not eating well.

Exercise is taboo also, I know. But there are ways. It's easy for me to say so, since I work at home (I'm a stay at home mom right now.), but it depends on how determined you were. I try to take a walk around the block once a day. I am not always successful. Sometimes I am just too tired. I have discovered I love yoga, but for right now, there are way too many poses that require being on the floor, stomach down, or chest strength that I just didn't have. It was a poor excuse, and I need to practice what I preach here. Exercising helps our physical, mental, and spiritual attitudes.

Find a place of peace. For me it was the woods, watching the animals frolic and chatter about. I love seeing the occasional deer walking through the back path. I could pray and see the wonders of God's hand; the mysteries of how it all works together.

Yesterday, I saw a hawk swoop down through the canopy of trees and grab something (a squirrel, I think), and swoop away again. I told a friend, and she said it was a sign of change. I responded in typical sarcastic fashion "so was I the hawk or the squirrel?" Either way, the biblical quote I have to say I live by the most is "Be still and know that I am God." (Psalm 46:10) I have had all sorts of fascinating things happen when I meditate on that scripture. I had found orphaned animals (which, as you know, I love to care for), or seen miracles of rainbows, or acts of unexpected kindness, or just the cleansing of the soul. God whispers, and we cannot hear him if we are always noisy.

God whispers, and we cannot hear him if we are always noisy.

No, the world does not go away when you are in stress. Sometimes it just keeps on piling up. I had some friends who do not have breast cancer, yet they were sick. One started chemotherapy day before yesterday; the other has been on a mild form of chemo for some time. As of yet, they still had their hair. For their sake, I hope they keep it. Losing your hair to chemo always seems like an insult to injury to me. But I could not let myself get stressed about them, because I still had my own health battles. That was not to say I didn't care, I just had to find a way to compartmentalize it all, do what I could, and let the rest go. It was challenging. It was time to go watch the rain come down, listen to the birds, and drink my second cup of coffee.

Find ways to enjoy your day. Good luck, I know you can do it!

Micro-chips

When you work in the veterinary field, you learn a lot of cool things. Many of them translate directly to the human medical field, but some were strictly meant for the animal field. One of those things that for now was strictly animal, but (to me) smacks of George Orwell's 1984, are microchips. Now, for those who do not know, these are little bitty microchips that are put under the skin using a needle to inject one, usually between the shoulder blades of an animal. It contains personal information about the animal, and there is a national database to help reunite owner and pet in event that the pet was lost. Ideally, it was a good thing considering how many pets got lost, and how few were ever found again. It reduces the number of pets put to sleep in shelters, when their owners simply had not been able to find them in time.

Well, a friend of mine got a new puppy. She has a ton of veterinary experience and runs a rescue group, so she does her own microchipping at home. I stopped by one day, because she had a new batch of cats come in very sick, and she needed to have the cages back that she had loaned me. She was having trouble wrangling a little poodle enough to both hold it still and give the shot with the microchip in it. Since the dog was so small, I figured I was strong enough now and could hold the pup while she put in the microchip.

Here's the scene. Small dog (smaller than my cats), being held in my arms against my chest, rather firmly so we could give the shot. Puppy was squirming and yelping like we were killing him, and I was holding firm. She presses in the needle, discharges the chip, and it dawns on me at that moment: If she missed the violently wriggling pup, and microchipped me instead, not only would I not feel it, but I would also pop and leak all over the place. So when we got done, she looked at me with wide fearful eyes, and asked, "Did we get it in the dog?" Then, of course we both laughed so hard I thought I was going to pee.

How would we explain that one to the plastic surgeon? "Um, yeah, I've popped my implant, but on a good note, I've been microchipped, so you can find me." Can you imagine the surgery to fix the implant? Where would the micro-chip be? Would they have to bring in the little hand-held device that locates and reads the chip? Would it be in the implant? Would it be embedded into some of the muscle? Just under the skin? This was killing me to think about, in a funny way, of course.

Now, what was really funny was that I just realized I've had a micro-chip in one breast before, but not the animal kind. The first time I found a lump in my breast (a bit over a year ago), they took a biopsy, then they put in a little titanium chip so that in future mammograms, they would know that at that spot, a biopsy had been done. Wait a minute, my memory was returning, I've had three. The first one, (which I just mentioned), was a "misfire" and they had to put a second chip in to make sure the first one got there, and then they put a third one in the spot where I did have cancer (on the other side). I found that amusing, considering we knew the whole breast would be removed anyhow.

Gotta love medical science!

Bathing Suits and Flapping in the Wind

I do not think I would be remiss in saying that one of the most dreaded things we as women do is buy bathing suits. We are critical of our bodies in the first place: "Do I look fat in this dress?"

So I'd say it's about tenfold worse when needing to buy a bathing suit. It was one those things that you tend to like to do in packs to get a more universal "Yes!" or "ummm…..no." Having to go alone was a very disconcerting thought, and for those of us not comfortable in our own skin (especially after a mastectomy), this can be downright scary.

Now, top all that off with a few things. First, it's the latter part of July. This translates to sale (good thing), but slim pickings (bad thing). Secondly: my condition. Now, I had the expanders in, which were now nicely pumped up enough to look semi normal. I personally think they look weird, but they pass enough for "normal" to buy a bathing suit and be seen in public. Maybe. The trick here was that I still hurt with any real pressure on the front, so spandex was not going to be my friend. Third: No underwire (OUCH!), since they were not … well … sitting normally yet (a bit too far apart). I couldn't have anything that expected the girls to be in their proper places.

So, off I went, alone, and admittedly scared to find a bathing suit. Now, the only reason I planned to torture myself was that I promised my sons that I would take them to a water park before school started, and I could not just go in regular clothes. I deserved to have some fun too. A friend suggested just wearing a tank top, which was a great idea, until I remembered they really stretch when wet.

Sigh.

So the search began. First thing I needed to do was to find my size. Now, my weight has fluctuated, my breast size was fluctuating (I truly had no idea where I was at since bras were too uncomfortable to wear, but I was assuming I was pretty close to where I was before), so I grab a few sizes to try on in the same styles that look like they might be comfortable and pretty. They were all separates, and the bottoms were not all exact matches to the tops, but they should be close enough to get away with. I figured halter-top types that could be adjusted were going to be my best bet. They all were pretty floral prints of some kind just like I always chose. At the last minute, I snagged one that just looked fun in leopard print. Every time I put on leopard print, I think it looks hideous, so I own nothing leopard print.

So, into the dressing room I go, and began to put on the six tops I found. They all either hurt, or showed my scars from one side or the other. By the time I was about done,

I was on the verge of tears. The bottoms oddly enough all fit, which was different, because that was usually my problem. So, I struggled not to cry, and I tried to decide if a tank top would just have to do as I was putting everything back on the hangers.

Yes, I know they pay people to do that, but to me it was a courtesy.

Then I spied the very last top, the leopard print. The style was different than all the others. Instead of the typical triangular shape of the cup, this top was more like a strapless top style, but with a halter tie. Hmm, at least I would hide the scars. The question was comfort. Most of them hurt getting on and off and then still hurt to wear, so I was less than optimistic.

I tried it on anyhow, and low and behold, it fit. Not only did it fit and hide the scars, but it was (GASP!) comfortable.

Yes, I had done it. I found a bathing suit for myself that I could wear even though I was still undergoing reconstruction. What a feat. So I went from tears to jumping for joy (I may have even shouted). The best part of all, it's modest enough to not embarrass my sons. OK, I'm their mom, so everything I do embarrasses them, but I thought it was pretty. So now I could go confidently to the water park.

I went from tears to jumping for joy.

Now, I spoke of the top, but I mentioned the bottom usually being the more difficult part of me to fit. This was true, as I found that most designer-cut suits to fit bottoms of women that had, well, how do I put it nicely? No shape. No shape to fall out the sides, no shape to creep into wedgies every time we bend over to retrieve something. I think the inventor of the thong was not trying to produce a sexier bikini, but I think he (or she) was a realist in that the bottom material was going to end up looking like that anyhow. May as well reduce the amount of material in there, and make it more comfortable and less of a hassle to constantly be pulling out.

That being said, women of my shape should not be wearing thongs in public in my opinion. I call them "butt floss." So when my alternatives feel like a choice between butt floss, and bottoms that creep up every step I take, it's going to feel like a losing battle. Good thing some kind soul invented skirt bottoms! That way you were covered.

Now, after buying my new suit (no butt floss for me), I went out to lunch with some friends to celebrate. Hey, this was huge for my ego! I got into the restaurant, and at first the air conditioning felt wonderful in contrast to the 104 heat index of the day. Then after about two beats, I was freezing. I decided if I was not going to shiver through lunch, I actually had to go get my sweater out of the car (how pathetic!). We were already in line, so I made a point to run to the car, since I parked a ways out.

As I was running, I realized two very important things. One, my new boobs were not moving (no bounce, shake, shimmy, or even a lift). The other thing I noticed was that my fanny was flapping away in the wind as if each cheek was waving good-bye to someone. Boy, was I glad I was not in that bathing suit, and made a new note to myself not to run at the water park, even if my life depended on it.

What do men think in these times? They like the bounce in the front. No more for me. Isn't the bounce in the back a bad thing? Women think so, don't men? So, now I had boobs tight enough to bounce a quarter off of (try it, and I will kill you), and a bottom that looks like Jell-O® (watch it wiggle, see it jiggle).

I was surprised that more women who do reconstruction do not insist on taking fat from their fannies to replace the fat in their breasts. Doctors don't do this simply out of logistical reasons (it was hard to get the right shape in either place afterward). Perhaps the surgeons should try harder to perfect this strategy. Perhaps when I donate my body to science when I die, it would be with the sole purpose of practicing getting the shape right for both bottom and top. I'd make sure I tell this to my plastic surgeon, and I'd also make sure to mention that in my will. Then again, they were welcome to take my fat now, and practice on someone else.

Somewhere in this time frame, and I do not remember when, I sat the boys down and wrecked their world.

"I'm leaving your dad."

I remember that Lee already knew this, Fred said he was expecting this and was kind of relieved we were finally talking about it. Alex was furious and crushed. His reaction startled me by his stating how worried he was about whether or not I was capable of caring for myself, both physically, and financially. He asked me to promise not to move out until I had at least recovered from my final implant surgery. I agreed, but the hunt for a place to live continued. I had begun to work on the idea for my business, and so I felt I would have a goal for finances. I had to find a place to live that was affordable, and preferably within walking distance of the house Lee would be living in. We had a rental house about a mile away from our current residence that he would be living in. I would not keep the boys from seeing Lee. He was gone enough with the military, so I was not going to limit the boys from seeing him when he was home. Even if that meant time they spent away from me.

See, I didn't hate Lee, I didn't think he was an awful person. I just couldn't get past my anger, hurt and disappointment of the times when he let me down. I was so afraid he would let me down again that I did not allow myself to see how wonderful he was in taking care of me at that moment as far as all the cancer stuff. You have to admit, this was better and more important than about anything else we had ever been through. However, I was not hearing any of it at that time. Ah, perspective. It changes everything.

Cry Here

One of the things about the hardships of life, cancer included, was that there were usually pivotal times in your life when you find out who your friends were and where they stand. It is amazing who leaves and who shows up to the party when it comes out that you have cancer or during any of the other pivotal times that are too numerous to mention. Some friends just kind of disappear, but others appear as if by magic out of the woodwork and give you more support than you ever would have expected or asked for. Most the time, it's both.

Although it was so thrilling to have the new ones appear, there was a definite blow in regards to those who disappear. There was this "what did I do?" mentality. Many times, it has nothing to do with me and everything to do with the other person, but it still leaves me questioning myself. I am a people pleaser. I like everyone to be happy, I like to make everyone happy, and I like everyone to like me. It's totally unrealistic, and I know that and I've matured a ton, but sometimes I still take it personally when I get blindsided by someone rejecting me that I thought I could count on.

Sometimes, what was going on with me was just too much for some people to handle (remember, we all have our own issues to deal with). Other times, I misinterpret the friendship and think there is more to it than there actually is. I'm sure there are friendships that I've strained by expecting too much from the other person. It's life, people. I know that, I've learned, and I've gotten over it.

Maybe it was less about me and the "who's there for me" issue, and more of the fact that every day, I was more and more convinced that I had started perimenopause, because my emotions were all over the place. I couldn't tell whether I was coming or going half the time. I would be sitting in an air conditioned room and feel hot (granted, I love that), or I would be outside on a warm day and feel like I was burning up. Some days, I just feel like curling up in a ball and bawling my eyes out, sometimes totally without reason.

Like yesterday for instance, I was driving home from somewhere, and this gal was running, and you could see her sports bra. No biggie. I thought to myself "Ha! I never have to wear one of those again!"

And then I immediately started crying.

Huh? I've always hated sports bras. They are uncomfortable, ugly, thick, and I was never sure whether you could wear them alone or were supposed to wear something over them (making them even bulkier). So why was I sitting there crying about never having to worry about something I didn't like anyhow? It was stupid. About as stupid as worrying about whether or not this person or that person liked me.

That is why I love my animals so much. You always know right where you stand. You feed them, they love you. Enough said. OK, I do believe there was so much more to it than that, but I never questioned where my pets would stand when I told them I was getting my boobs chopped off. The only thing that mattered to them was that they could no longer use them as their personal pillows. They adapted, they adjusted (as do I), and found another spot to lie down and be comfy.

Another thing I learned was that there were more fair weather friends than foul weather friends. More people were there for you to laugh and have fun with, but there were few who were willing to let you cry with them. I was watching a country song video, and I cannot for the life of me remember which one. There was a guy in the video with a tattoo on his shoulder that had an arrow pointing to the top of his shoulder and writing underneath that said "cry here." I loved that tattoo, and there was a part of me that dearly wished I knew that guy and that he would let me cry on his shoulder, too. I would love to chalk it all up to menopause-type stuff, because I knew that I would be fine.

Wait a minute, I forgot the surgery to take out the ovaries was still ahead, and then it would be really bad for a while. Oh, crap. Either way, I'd be OK, and I'll soldier through it all. I may not have the good "stiff upper lip" like the English, but I would make it and be OK. Not sure my sons would. They may need some serious therapy.

On the note of needing someone to cry with, I needed to buy a case of wine (or something), because another friend of mine was going through her own version of hell. Her hubby kept having these heart attacks (he's my age at about forty and had his eighth heart attack this month), and they couldn't seem to really control them. I could see it was wearing on her. Perhaps we could have a good cry together. I better give her a call. Misery loves company, and now I understand why.

Loss of a Family Member

I sit here at my computer feeling empty. As I had mentioned several times, there was more out there than just cancer. My sister-in-law, Cynthia, lost her battle with multiple sclerosis yesterday. Soon I would be flying out to Arizona for the funeral. How could I handle this? It's so hard to be happy that I'm alive and going to be OK, when my family has just lost a loved one. How could I rejoice that my treatments were coming to an end when other family members were suffering? There was something about it all that seemed inherently wrong.

Of course it's wrong. We die. It sucks, and it's totally out of our control.

When I had my surgery and got the infection, my sister-in-law was already on a feeding tube, and the feeding tube became infected. She had to have a PICC line put in, same as me. Only then she got blood clots and other infections, and just plain went downhill from there.

I talked to her quite a bit, but not daily. I spoke with my brother to see how he was doing, and I got the typical "we've been down this road before, we're fine." Which,

I didn't buy, but he's so far away, I couldn't tell how he was doing. One of the things about our family was that we were stronger than we should have to be and always have been.

There had been many rifts in the family in the more recent years for many reasons, but I was praying perhaps, somehow, someway, by some miracle, they could be healed a bit with our grieving. I needed my family, and I had always known that. The rifts were terrible, but not all of them were things I could fix. Some of them I did have some responsibility for, but others I had to leave be. I know so many of you reading this are in similar boats. You know what this means, and how hard it can be to move forward based on what has passed.

Knowing I had to get on a plane did not help either. I no longer like to fly. It scares me. I have experienced plenty of nasty flight attendants, and I am phobic of the sensation of turbulence. We paid extra and got nonstop flights. Less boarding, fewer takeoffs and landings, and fewer flight attendants.

Today, the boys and I went shopping for appropriate clothing for the upcoming occasion. The boys' church that was walking distance from the house, and different from mine, was very casual, so they had no "church" clothes. I needed to figure out what I could comfortably wear. I felt like all this weight was upon me. I knew how to de-stress, but it was not lifting that weight. Honestly, I was too tired to bother. I'd rather have gone back to bed.

Cancer took a piece (or two) of me, but multiple sclerosis took my sister-in-law slowly, agonizingly, and over many years. She was finally at peace, she could walk, she could dance, she could run (I never ever saw her run). She was finally pain free with no more needles, no more tests, no more tubes.

She was in the loving hands of God. That could be celebrated. I prayed for my brother and nephew who had been her total caretakers for years. They had no more tubes to change, wounds to check, special meals to fix or infinite doctor appointments to go to. This changed how their world had been for years. I prayed for God's peace for them in the new life ahead of them. I loved them, I worried about them, and I knew that in time they would be OK.

The right words for support seem to always evade me. I never seem to feel as if I had said the right thing. I try to imagine what people would say to me, and to me anything was OK, but I knew that they might need to be hearing something different. Sometimes the best thing was to say nothing at all, but to cry with them instead. That, I knew I could do.

Places

One of the places I find to be the most peaceful is the beach with the crashing waves of the ocean and the noise of the seagulls. The other place I find to be the most peaceful are the woods in the early morning with all of their sounds. So, when people ask me if I am a mountain or an ocean person, I truly have a hard time answering. There is much healing for me in both.

The overwhelming, relentless crashing of the waves never cease to remind me how small I am and that no matter how big my burdens, even they are small in the grand scheme of life. To me, that perspective is helpful, soulful, and gives me assurance that I can get through anything. I imagine all my burdens being tossed into those waves and having them being beaten back, beaten down, and destroyed. I feel as if I am watching a battle of my emotions being waged in those waves, and the sights, sounds, and sensations are proof that I will be OK.

The morning sounds of the forest on the other hand, are soft (generally) and greet me with a renewed sense of life. I find myself able to concentrate and listen carefully to all the different noises. How many types of birds are there this morning? What animals are stirring or going to sleep? It was not quite dawn and so the crickets and cicadas continue softly, quietly, sleepily, while I was arousing groggily to shuffle down, feed the wailing animals (you know, the loud, demanding cats), make my coffee, open the deck door, listen to the sounds of the world, and awaken. Sometimes (often now), I find myself awakening to the sounds of my fingers on the keyboard as I process things in my head that kept me up the night before.

I love watching the leaves seem to come alive as the sun touches the tops of them and ever so slowly move down. I enjoy the glistening of the spider webs that seem to dance between the branches in the filtering sunlight. Occasionally, I get the joy of watching a deer go sauntering past along the trail outside my fence.

I get to watch the glory of one of God's new days, the only today He would ever make. What would it be like? I never know. It could be as beautiful as the safe and timely arrival of a baby or as devastating as the loss of a loved one. Either way, outside of ourselves there is peace all around us.

Perhaps I just need a place with a babbling brook and the woods. Anyone know of a cabin or house for sale fitting that description?

Finding peace, somehow and somewhere, is paramount to surviving anything thrown at you. I cannot imagine how difficult finding that bit of peace in a war zone would be with the constant threat of danger and ever presence of violence. And yet, there was peace to be found.

One of the reasons I wanted to go live in South Korea for the time we were stationed there, was because I wanted to understand how those people, that country, lived each day knowing their greatest enemy was like a poised tiger waiting for a moment of weakness to strike and always living right at their back door. South Korea is a peninsula. North Korea is their only bordering country. There is no secret that North Korea is a constant threat. So, how do the people live under that looming shadow? Do they cower in fear? Are they jumpy and constantly looking over their shoulders?

No. I was amazed at their resilience, and amazed at the graciousness of their culture. Imagine a city with the size and population of New York City, without all the crime, and safe enough to go anywhere in the city, day or night, in total safety (OK, there was the occasional pick pocket, but that was about it). If there was a problem, someone would try to help you. It's not like big cities here, where they ignore you as if you do not exist. They interact, they respond. No, you don't say hi to everyone, or even say excuse me when you constantly bump into people, but they are nice, they smile, they converse with you. It's just different. They had found a peace.

In times of war, there are ways to find peace. The reasons I think they have such a peace is not only because of the traditions, but the religions. Remember, the largest single church population in the world, Presbyterian, was located in Seoul, South Korea. I got to hear stories of miraculous rescues attributed to Angels of God, and I believe them. I heard stories of finding peace, even if only within themselves: While hunkering down in a hut while being bombed, they knew that they really would be OK. And they believed and they were not afraid.

That was peace.

The Tape Won't Break

I remember when I was in high school, which was a particularly stressful and sad time in my life, I reached a point one night, where everything that had gone wrong in the last three years just seemed to be overwhelming me and hit me over head with the stupidest thing: tape. Simple, stupid Scotch tape. Or so I thought. I was working on a project for my debate class that I was not confident about simply because it was the first time I had done it.

I had everything cut out, and it was due to be used the next day at my first debate tournament. Taping the notes to the cards was the last thing I had to do. I was not procrastinating, but I was nervous. All the other stress was weighing there too (I always seemed to be stressed in those days). I was trying to get the Scotch tape to simply tear off of the roll, like any normal tape was supposed to do yet it was not working. Now, it turned out to be a special clear thin packing tape that required scissors (it had been put on one of those cute little rollers ladies use in their offices when I was trying to use it). But between being so nervous about my first tournament, and trying to accomplish this supposedly simple task, and all the stress at the time, I started bawling and bawling. I called one of my friends (who will no doubt read this and comment) and cried into the phone "The tape won't break!"

Of course, bless her heart, that statement made absolutely no sense to her whatsoever. But she knew I was really upset, and that was all that mattered. She came over immediately, and we talked and figured out the stupid tape was not the normal kind, and therefore, I was not as incapable as I certainly was feeling.

So when things overwhelm me, and that one stupid little thing that is really so easy becomes impossible to accomplish, I start thinking, "The stupid tape won't break!" I know it was just a lot of things hitting me at once that were all too much to tackle, and I'd had no choice but to just do the next thing. But then, when doing the next thing results in something breaking, suddenly making things even more difficult, I throw my hands up.

I was having one of those mornings…

One of the removable little plastic parts of my refrigerator was dirty. No problem, I could remove it, wash it, and return it. Simple. So, as I was trying to pull that out, I bumped the shelf above it, and it totally collapsed on me. Crap! I took a good look at it and realized I had managed to break a piece on the door, kind of like a button, that was smaller than my pinkie nail. We were not talking a removable piece that I could take out and replace. It was something on the door-side. You know, that part that is connected to the solid plastic piece that makes up the inside door of my fridge. Great! I didn't think super glue worked under refrigerated conditions, but I guess we were going to find out.

This was not in my plans for today. Today, I was supposed to be painting all of the stupid storage closets. Now I was ticked (and writing, which I was also not planning on because I wanted to finish the painting today), and had to waste Lord only knows how much time to fix the fridge.

Actually, no, I did not.

All the food was still able to go into the fridge, and the shelf that was broken was not necessary at the moment. I'd just put it aside, and leave it under the "to-do" list.

That relieved stress already.

When things go wrong for me, I have this impulsive internal expectation to fix it immediately, as if neglecting to do so would result in the world collapsing or at the least the house. So, sometimes it is difficult for me to let go of things that happen, and leave them for later, and know that it be OK. This is especially true, when so many other things going on around me were one hundred percent out of my control. I want to fix, I want to rescue, and I want everything and everyone to be OK all the time. But this is not reality, as nice as it would be.

A friend and I were talking on the phone early today, because the local humane society was so packed with cats they were (get this) *giving* them away! Already spayed or neutered, with their shots, microchipped, and free. Now, I am not a hoarder, but I can enjoy a larger than normal number of cats, and love it, and keep them happy, healthy, and very well cared for. However, I had enough cats, and the only thing keeping me from getting "just one more" was the knowledge that I would not be able to afford it should anything major go wrong.

I have this personal policy that I live by when it comes to pets, partly learned by experience, partly by training. I would never own so many animals that if something traumatic (translate expensive) happened to more than one animal or if the whole house got sick at once, that I could not afford to care for them. I was comfortably at that limit now. I would not push it.

But I wanted to rescue something. I wanted the house to quit breaking. I wanted people I loved to quit getting sick or die. I wanted the world to be at peace so families did not have to be ripped apart by wars. I wanted the Garden of Eden.

That was not going to happen anytime soon or at least not soon enough for me. That's life, and I knew that. Sometimes it's just frustrating, and it gets to all of us sometimes. It's one of those times for me this morning, but I would go put on old clothes and take another step into putting my life back together. I vented, I was good, I would move on. I would paint.

Like Buying a Car

I admit that it never occurred to me that the exact amounts of saline or silicone in the final implants were of such importance, until one of my friends explained it to me. She kept asking exactly how much I had in now, and I kept responding with "around such-n-such." She finally said, "Sarah, you aren't listening. This is like buying a car, only different."

Really?

Really, really. Apparently, I would get a bunch of paperwork that stated exactly how much saline or silicone was in each side, and I would have special registration numbers and all sorts of fun stuff. I had more research ahead. I did not know this. I would get, not VIN numbers, but rather PIN numbers (Prosthetic Identification Numbers).

Now I was being silly here, but these numbers, whatever they were actually called, were going to be very important and needed to be registered. Part of all this I did not yet understand. Part of it was so that the company that manufactured the implants could keep track of everyone in case it turned out that a batch that was recalled. Then I would be notified and fast.

After a bit of preliminary research, I discovered the registration was not for the company to keep track of, but for me to keep track of. The company publishes what numbers may be affected, and it would be up to me (and the registry?) to know if my numbers were included. My doctors, the company, and about everyone (possibly including me), would eventually forget not only the registration numbers, but how much was in them. But since this information was as important as knowing the square footage of your house, I had to keep it some place safe.

Yesterday, I went to the grocery store after my fill and just picked up a few things. It was so nice to be able to go to the store unassisted and do my shopping, even if it wasn't much. As I was unloading the cart, it began to roll away from me. Instinctively, I grabbed for it with my left hand, which was the same side I had the infection. When I did, I had a horrible shooting pain in my shoulder and down my arm. I couldn't believe it. I'd injured myself reaching for a stupid runaway shopping cart. This would seriously delay my healing, especially since no one could believe I had actually injured myself that way.

My head was fuzzy this morning. Between hurting my shoulder and this last fill I got yesterday, I needed the heavy stuff, so I took some codeine last night. I took the lesser amount but should have taken the larger dose, because I didn't sleep so well. Oh well. It was all part of the process.

The Toughest Stuff

I find myself having trouble writing, because the passing of my sister-in-law tripped off some unresolved grief in a different area of my life. You know, the type of grief that was so painful that you could only take it in small doses, like dipping your foot in the pool to test the waters.

Then something seems to come along and push you head-long into the pool. I had not mentioned this issue much before, because it was too painful to bring up. However, now it was once again brought to the forefront for me, and was worth explaining.

I was still grieving terribly for the loss of my daughter and the loss of all the dreams I had for her to have a wonderful life. They were all gone. The daughter I loved and tried to save was no longer mine to have. Yet, because the courts had not yet let things be done, my grief could not be completed. I was stuck in limbo.

I would get no mark of the passing of this relationship. No funeral as if she had died, no loving family flying in to help me grieve and let me know I was loved and that they knew I tried my best. I never would get that.

And, right now, that hurt. I was grieving the loss of my child alone. My sons, having been terrorized by her, never shed a tear at her leaving and were glad and relieved she was gone. They were safe again. They no longer loved her. They did not understand my tears and how hard it all was. They did not understand it would always be hard.

Since the situation with my daughter caused so much of the tribulation in my marriage, the last place I felt I could go for comfort was to my husband. I did not feel supported by him. I blamed him for a lot of what transpired. I felt that there was no way I could depend on him at that time. Especially not for this grief.

They say that stress is a contributing factor to getting cancer. Imagine that. So it was no wonder to me at all that my cancer would develop now of all times. But I could not handle it all at once. No one could. So I went from moment to moment, day to day. I was doing amazingly well, considering.

TSA

About the time I flew to Arizona for Cynthia's funeral, there was a big hubbub about TSA and the screenings. Later, there was also a huge uproar about screenings for breast cancer survivors. I had those screenings, and I wish to add my two bits.

Now, I had hurt my shoulder, and I had hurt it more than I knew even at the time. In fact, I was in pain from that July 2010 up until April 2011. At the time of my flight, I was in so much pain that I could not lift my arm. I was picked for the x-ray, and I was told to put my arms above my head and hold them there.

Excuse me? You want me to do WHAT? I could not. I truly, physically, simply could not. And I told them so.

> Excuse me? You want me to do WHAT?

Of course, per protocol, they then had to do a pat down. I asked if I could have the pat down in private, and I had a feeling they would find that the implants were, well, not normal. The implants look, and feel abnormal, and in this day and age of terrorists on planes, I didn't blame them for checking me out. I was grateful my dad was travelling with me and the boys. Lee was still deployed, of course. I told the boys I would be right back and to just stay with Grandpa. When we got to the private room, I told the gals I had breast cancer, that I was in the middle of reconstruction, and that I had hurt my shoulder. I knew that when they felt the implants (no, I was not totally felt up), that they might feel the need to check things out more thoroughly. No, I didn't appreciate being checked out, but think of it this way; don't you want to make sure the other guy next to you was truly not a terrorist? After all, you don't know him. For the other passengers, I was the other guy.

As I had mentioned already, I had travelled. I was also aware that a large number of people had not travelled outside of US borders. On that note, and my answer to the complaints about TSA: deal. What would you rather have? Two ladies politely and apologetically giving you a pat down or would you rather have guards armed with assault rifles aimed at you asking you to strip right there in the waiting area? That is what happens in some foreign countries when they do screenings. We forget how good we have it. As far as being searched, our TSA guys (and gals), are the politest, most considerate of any agency I have ever been searched by.

I also discovered that they often search people based on two factors: those they think might actually pose a threat and those who seem to be the nicest and most forgiving about being pulling aside to be searched. Now, I imagine if you were just plain being a snot to everyone around you, I could understand how they might like to make your day just a bit worse. We all love to see the jerks get put in their places. The TSA are doing their best to assess real risks in a thankless job, in a hostile, threatening environment, and they try to do so nicely and patiently. I am not saying they are perfect or that they are always polite. Think about it, would you want their job? I have heard that the TSA is considering allowing people with medical disabilities, or anything that TSA might find abnormal, to carry a medical card stating the issue. In the case of breast cancer patients, they would be aware that perhaps a gal has prosthetics. I like the idea of the medical cards to avoid embarrassing pat downs.

That being said: Give them a break, or perhaps they will start taking lessons from other countries and start asking to search you at gunpoint. Take your pick.

In Memory of Cynthia

Well, one of the rougher weekends of my life was finally over. My sister-in-law's services were beautiful and done as a celebration of life as opposed to a mourning of her passing, because she had been so sick and in pain for so long.

My brother managed to pull together a slide show of pictures of her from years past, and many of them I remembered. I had known her for, let me think here a minute: just shy of thirty years of my life. While watching the slide show, I was most struck by one of her wedding pictures that I remembered and loved. I did not have a copy of this particular picture, so I had totally forgotten about it until there it was, up on the screen. It was all of us bridesmaids holding our bouquets around her face, such that it was framed. It was gorgeous. It was my favorite picture of their wedding.

I saw her mom there, knowing that Cynthia was her only child, and thought how wrong it was to outlive your children, regardless of how old they were. I knew she had step brothers, but I do not believe any of them were there. I never met them. We were all there from our side.

I remember I was so nasty to her when I first met her. I was terribly jealous of her, and I knew that she knew. I was quite a bit younger than she was. I was a pre-teen, and she was in her early twenties. My brother Rich had been a huge part of my life. I was losing him and could not view it as gaining her: wasn't happening. I remember we were sitting around the house talking, and one of the typical family sayings would come up and I would always glare at her, arms tightly folded across my chest and say, "We say things like that in THIS family."

Oh, was I a pill.

But I remember her taking me roller skating and sometimes out shopping, although I could not for the life of me remember where we went, aside from getting ice cream. She tried to be nice at a time when I wasn't really happy about it all. She still invited me to be in the wedding.

I remember my bridesmaid dress. Mom made it from the pattern that Cynthia had picked out. To try out the pattern, she made a dress first out of an old bed sheet of mine. It was cute, but definitely too low cut for a young girl with AAA-cup size (with room to spare). So Mom adjusted the bodice upwards about two inches to accommodate. I remember that I even wore the "bed sheet dress" to a dance at school. I was in junior high then. I had a picture of that dress somewhere. I may have to find it.

Cynthia had unbelievably dry wit that was very fast, and she loved an argument for the sake of an argument sometimes. I really never got to know her well enough to understand quite where I stood. My parents and I moved out of state not long after they were married. I would forever be the little sister. I know that. My brothers haven't really gotten to know me as an adult, and I know that. Part of the hazard of the military lifestyle is that it is hard to maintain family relationships when you are not close by and can't visit regularly.

I do have to mention something that she would probably be a bit angry with me for, but it really hit me in a positive way. She always dressed to the nines. She always had her hair fixed, make up on, beautiful clothes, nails manicured and painted, all the accessories, and she had nice perfume on always, always, always. She was also overweight. Now, the reason I mention these things together (I hope you understand and forgive me, Cynthia), was that she taught me that there was no excuse for not looking your best. So many people that are overweight do not care about their appearance. They wear poorly fitting clothes. They don't wear make up properly (women, of course), and I have known more than my fair share of them that do not wear good deodorant, or perfumes, or colognes. Many people are overweight, and treated poorly not just because they are overweight, but because they do not care for themselves. She never lacked for self-esteem. She took care of her appearance. She was always beautiful and smelled good. She was always prettier than me. It didn't matter who was thinner. She was beautiful, she knew it, and it showed.

Many people in the world I am in now are prejudice against overweight people, and have many misconceptions about them. Thanks to Cynthia, I never had that. I could always see that they had the inner beauty, but the individual chose whether or not to show the outer beauty. I was always able to tell those people making snide remarks that not all people who are overweight look baggy. Not all overweight people smell badly. Not all overweight people "look awful." I knew one that was always beautiful.

I always wondered what she really thought of me until about a year or two ago. I had some very trying times in my life, where a difficult situation had arisen that only part of the story was told and rumors flew. I was getting bashed right and left by people who believed the rumors, as opposed to asking me about the situation, or just knowing the truth by my character (which I always thought was above question, but I guess that was wrong). She did something unexpected for me. She did something very few others in my life did. She very vocally stood up for me and dispelled the rumors. She said she knew me well enough to know that I would never do what the rumors said I had done and how dare anyone even question that, as I had never even remotely behaved in a manner that would indicate anything other than pure motives.

I was floored and thrilled. She was so vocal, that many of the rumors stopped cold. No, she was not the only one, but she was the loudest, and the most unexpected source, and I will be forever grateful to her for that gift of protection and faith in me.

We talked a lot more often towards the end. She knew that I understood a lot of the medical stuff going on in her life, and she knew what it was like to be sick for a long time and in pain all the time. We had very different diseases, but that part of our lives was a real connection of understanding. We especially bonded when it came to our PICC line experiences.

About a week after I got my PICC line, I got a call from her. By this time in her progression of multiple sclerosis, she was on a stomach tube for feeding and it had become infected. So, lucky her, she got a PICC line, too. She called because hers hurt terribly, and she wanted to know if I was having the same experience. I told her that, no, mine was actually painless. We compared notes, and discovered that hers had been placed too low on her arm, too close to her elbow, and too close to a nerve. Her arm hurt so badly she couldn't lift it. Soon afterward, because of not being able to move it, she got a massive blood clot in her shoulder. Not good.

They removed that PICC line and put one in the other arm. That one did not hurt, and was well placed. Unfortunately, that one got infected as well, and so on and so on. They never were able to get her infections cleared up, and they probably reached her heart, causing the heart attack that took her life.

It was agonizing to see my brother grieve, and I found myself unable to hold back own tears of grief for them and their son, who although grown up, had still lost his mom. My nephew never got the opportunity to have a mom well enough to be a typical soccer mom, but I knew she did her best, and he was a good person who seemed grounded in his faith, and he would be all right.

My brother was out of work for almost two years, and was her caretaker 24/7. Three hundred sixty-five days a year. She was his entire world. I worried for him now that she was gone. I knew he had plans, things he could now do. I knew he was relieved to no longer have to worry about how she was, if she was OK, or if she needed him. I knew it was nice for him to think about getting to travel again; something he had not been able to freely do in years. He was a fabulous husband to her, taking care of every need, sacrificing everything for her. He was the type of husband every woman wants; one that she knew would lay down his life for hers, and he pretty much did just that. Always making sure she came before anything else.

One of the reasons he had trouble finding work was that no one was flexible enough to realize that he needed to be able to leave at the drop of a hat if something was wrong at home. They needed to understand that she couldn't leave her bed, couldn't feed herself, and could hardly roll over unassisted in her weakness. He did not make enough money to afford a full-time nurse, and they really didn't want one. He wanted to take care of her, and he did.

Until the end.

As Christ loved the church and laid down His life for her, my brother put aside his own life for the remaining time they had together. Now, he got to go on and had his life, but without her, it would still be hard.

They had a marriage that you dream of. They never argued. They occasionally disagreed, but never argued. I am not sure how they managed that one, since Cynthia loved to argue for the sake of an argument. Things may not have always been as smooth with other relationships within the family, but that didn't matter. They were happy, and that was how it should be.

I wish we all could have been as lucky. It seemed unfair that such a wonderful marriage had to end so soon. Those are the ones that deserve to go on forever as an example to the rest of us on how to do it.

I needed to go to PT. It was time to get back to living my life and do the day to day again. Life goes on, the sun comes up in the east and sets in the west, and the birds are singing in the trees.   I was thankful I had today. It was time to go live it.

OK to Not be OK

Sometimes, it's OK to not be OK. I found it frustrating that when I was at my sister-in-laws funeral and I was crying, everyone kept asking if I was OK.

No, I was not OK.

Of course I said I was. What were they going to do if I said I wasn't OK? Why was it not OK to be sad? Why was it not OK to have a hard time when so much stress was going on in my life? Why do I always have to be OK? Why couldn't it be OK to be grieving, tired, sad, hurting, frustrated, and just plain not OK? It didn't mean I would always be not OK, nor did it mean I was going to do anything stupid. Yes, things were difficult. I was going through a lot, but I was not suicidal, people.

There was more going on in my life than just the cancer, and everything was compounded by the shoulder injury, and the passing of a family member. You know those stress indicator tests you can take? You know, the ones where they give point values to things like moving, death or divorce of a spouse or family member, changing jobs, etc. You add up those numbers and it gives you an indicator of your stress level. I found that puppy and calculated mine.

It said that anyone with a score over 300 would become ill from immunity issues caused by stress (like, oh, I don't know... cancer?). My score? 451. Now, that included my immunity issue that I already was dealing with caused by the rest of that 451.

Why do I always have to be OK?

Was I worried? No. I was not. Why? Because it's OK to not be OK when there is that much stress in your life.

It's time to learn to relax, breathe deeply, and accept that you are just along for the ride. I had faith that God had a plan for me. There was a reason for all of it. But that didn't mean I would ever know, nor understand that plan. It just meant that He was in control, and I was not.

Not by a long shot. They say the only one you can control is yourself, and I find myself having trouble doing that. I shouldn't be trying to control anyone else when I can't control myself or even my mouth.

What a relief it is to not be responsible for anyone else's actions or choices! We have a responsibility for our own actions and how those affect others, but we are not responsible for their actions. How nice is that? I don't have to worry about it.

My oldest son, Fred, was getting his braces off today. He should have gotten them off a year ago, but he wouldn't wear the rubber bands. At almost sixteen, I did not feel it was any longer my responsibility to harp on him about it. He was old enough.

The consequence of his actions: He had the braces on until he chose to do something about it.

The assistants at the dentist office would tell me I had to check him to make sure he was wearing the bands. I told them, no, I did not. If he wanted to get married with his braces on, that was his choice. Eventually, he got the point. He started wearing his rubber bands, and today, he gets his braces off.

Good for him!

Not my responsibility to make him do anything. I can influence him, but I should not stress about my part in his choices; they were his to screw up, or do to the letter of instruction. That was his choice. I would not take it from him.

Along the same lines, my younger son, Alex, was a freshman in football, and he was the smallest on the team. I fretted for him and his safety. I also wanted to stay well informed. He didn't want an over-protective mom hanging around. He wanted to do it himself, and he was capable of doing a good job of it. I just found it difficult to let go and let him. My responsibility of doing things for him was getting smaller at light speed, and I needed to let it.

That was stressful too. At the same time, it was awesome! It sure simplified my life. He's making good choices and doing a good job. They both were. If they needed something, they would come to me. It was time to give them more control over their own reins and just sit beside them on the ride.

My role as a parent was changing. The good thing was that really did free me up to start really taking care of myself, which I had never really done. I got to start thinking about what I wanted to do. I chose to have my kids young and be a stay at home mom. I had no regrets.

Soon, though, it would be my turn. They no longer needed me for much more than as a taxi these days, as far as real care. They could fix their own meals, wipe their own bottoms, and tie their own shoes. They were at school, and I do not have to be at home sitting by the phone waiting to be needed.

Even when they have a cold, there was no longer much for me to do. I care take because that was what I was programmed to do. But I do not really need to anymore. They can do it for themselves. I know they appreciated it, and I liked to do it. Soon, they would be living somewhere else, and they would do it for themselves.

Stress comes and goes, that was part of life. Sometimes, it feels like a bully ganging up on you and beating you within an inch of your life. Then it was my choice to get up again and again, as often as it takes, and go on. I could learn how to avoid certain stressors and learn to deal with others. I could learn how to pray deeper, relax more, and appreciate life.

I saw a funny video that really has more to it than the silliness of it. It was called the Gratitude Dance. It was a goofy little dance that a bunch of people were doing, but the point was to be grateful for things. No matter how bad it may get in your life, there was always something to be grateful for. There was always a reason to smile, even in the midst of tears.

I was being shaped like a diamond. Sounded good to me. I was being polished, cut, and shaped, and it was a painful process. I had to go from a seeming lump of coal and be compressed, heated, dug up, and then made into the beautiful, clear shiny stone that we equate with love. Diamond is one of the hardest substances on earth. Why do you think there is such a thing as a diamond-tipped drill bit for metal? You are free to equate that hardness to my stubbornness, although I prefer the term perseverance. They are the same thing.

Perseverance just sounds more like a quality rather than a fault. Either way, I'm hard as stone, baby.

Or perhaps like a rose. Did you know that to make roses really grow well, they require pruning? Not just a bit here and there, but at the end of the season, you hack it off at the base.

Ouch.

But then you cover it to protect it from the winter to come, and in the spring, you have a bigger, stronger, more beautiful rose bush than the previous year. I've been hacked back. Right now, I was being covered (I view that as covered in prayer and faith in God's love), and it was time for me to rest until spring.

Let's go got those braces off. It was another important day in my son's life. I was happy and grateful to be a part of it.

Women of High Profile

I had an appointment with my plastic surgeon last Friday. It was really eye opening. Eye popping, really. I'm sitting there in the room, in the all too familiar gown open to the front, and he walks in with this tub of prosthetic breast implants. They were a variety of shapes and sizes, about ten of them.

Holy cow! Really?

The different shapes had to do not only with the amount of milliliters in each, but the width of your chest wall, as well. As it would happen, I needed the smallest width for my chest wall. You would think that with that narrow of a chest wall that I would have as much as I do in each expander and still look normal – not like Anna Nicole Smith or something. I'm still scratching my head over that one.

So, I was going to need the narrowest implants, which were called "high profile." I could see how they were going to certainly make a bigger impact in that they were about the size and shape of a grapefruit. The others were shaped more like a huge M&M, and were too wide. If I had gotten those they would have met in the middle and wrapped around under my arms. Yet, I would think that it would reduce the cup size. My doctor said not really. I'm still trying to wrap my brain around that one. Maybe it has more to do with chest width then than cup size or shape. I'll be going someplace that does real bra fittings and finding a nice lady to help me figure out what the cup size would be with these new projecting boobs.

There was a Women of Faith conference in my area this weekend, and I definitely went. I always find myself held accountable, uplifted, humbled, and encouraged at these. I always discover something new about myself, and usually come home with a love for a new musical talent. This time was no exception. To me, the most profound moment was when one of the musicians spoke about losing his daughter at birth. He asked all those who had lost a child to stand. I was amazed and saddened to see the sheer number of women who stood. Oh, the tears that flowed. Such grief they all could share, knowing they were not alone by any stretch.

I wondered if others would really count me among them.

I stood, but I wondered if others would really count me among them.

They had speakers who were abused, had eating disorders, broken homes, lost children, and been widowed. Some speakers had recently become mothers, had great marriages, and had incredible talents singing or performing abilities. But, I felt there was one thing missing: a cancer veteran. No one had talked about fighting and surviving cancer. It takes incredible strength to fight cancer, solid faith and humor were the two main factors in indicating survival. They need someone to talk about that experience. I actually think I am going to write them about that. Should I volunteer?

I had a dream a few months ago, a very weird one. I do not remember it completely, but what I do remember was that upon waking up, I was very clearly told to "tell Sheila."

Sheila? Sheila Walsh? Author, singer, and Women of Faith speaker? Really?

Tell her what? I had no idea. I didn't have one thing of hers. I like her music, but didn't own any of it. I did not have any of her books at that point. I had no reason to be thinking of her at all.

However, I wrote a letter and told her...

Well, I told her I had a nudging to write her, but no idea what I was supposed to tell her, or why. What a screwy letter it was! But I sent it. I did not expect to get a response, and I had not.

When I was at the Women of Faith conference, she was there. She was only doing a book signing on Friday during lunch, which I missed, and also first thing Saturday morning. I was the driver for several people, so I could not get there early, but I did my best. As I walked in the direction she was doing the signing, I realized I had nothing for her to sign, and I didn't know if she had even gotten my letter. I wasn't about to go up empty handed and expect her to have a clue who I was. I stopped to buy a book. That took all of about a minute. I got into the back of the long line to meet her and waited.

I didn't have to wait long before a lady came along, and stopped and said "I'm sorry. We have to cut off the line now." They stopped the line three people in front of me. I guess I was not meant to get that opportunity.

Alright. I admit it leaves me still wondering why or what I was supposed to tell her. I guess I will never know.

Today was the first day of school for my younger son. He's a freshman at the local high school. He's ready. I had faith that he would make good choices. The high school has the first day of school specifically for freshman alone, so they have time to get their bearings and find their classes before the rest of the students arrive the next day. It's a good opportunity to meet the other freshman, find their lockers and classes, and meet their teachers. My older son survived it, and could hardly wait until the second day, which he calls "freshman kill day" just to be intimidating. It wasn't working. I couldn't believe they were both in high school now. I got an incredible amount of satisfaction in that, because they were awesome boys with morals and solid heads. They made good choices most of the time and chose good friends.

Again, my days would be free. It was not that summer wasn't free, but being a stay at home mom for so long kind of left me with this mind set of needing to be at home, as if they still needed me all the time. I didn't stay at home all day or anything, but by not working, I was not committed to anything that I could not drop immediately and go take care of my boys.

Cats and Rimadyl Do Not Mix

I felt as if I was in a downward spiral. Falling, as if the rope I tied the knot in to hang on has failed. I felt overwhelmed, anxious, frustrated, exhausted, confused, and just plain all around not OK.

My routine in the morning was always to get up, use the potty, feed the cats, go downstairs, feed the dog, feed the birds, get my coffee, and then get on the computer. It's my routine.

Well, now my dog has arthritis and takes a medication called Rimadyl. He takes a 100 mg tablet that was beef flavored and very tasty to him. He was still upstairs in my son's room when I put his food in his bowl, so I put his medication right on top. I fixed my coffee, which consists of a cup of microwaved hot water and instant coffee. I turned around, and there was Charcoal, our short-haired, overweight, eighteen-month-old black cat, sitting and eating the dog's food. So I looked, and sure enough, the little stinker ate the Rimadyl. That's a problem.

Rimadyl was not for cats, even at a cat-sized dose, which would be about 7 mg for him. He ate 100 mg. This was bad, very bad. This was at 0600 in the morning. I did what I knew to do, which was to give him hydrogen peroxide, to try to get him to throw up. It didn't work. So there Charcoal and I sat, in the bathroom until about 0715. We got him to the vet by the time they opened at 0730 on the dot, and they took over. Long story short, he seemed to be fine, but we still would not know for sure for another week.

The last thing I needed was to lose one of my beloved cats. This one was attached to my son Fred and to our dog. This cat had dumb luck. Well, he was a black cat, after all.

He made his mark on the staff of the veterinarians' office we were in for two reasons: The first was that he hates going to the vet. He screams and fights and is in general not a pleasant or cooperative cat to work with. He is not one of their preferred clients.

The second reason he left his mark had to do with this particular visit. One of the treatments for accidental poisoning was to give liquid activated charcoal. It binds with the poison in the stomach, does not allow the body to absorb it, and then passes harmlessly out the other end.

So, they were giving Charcoal charcoal. It struck everyone as funny. This was even more so with the administration of said product. The feisty brute got charcoal everywhere: all over the technicians trying to administer it, all over the table, floor, and all over the cat himself. Well, he was a black cat, covered in black liquid charcoal. They couldn't see it on him to clean it off, so the poor beast got charcoal all over everything for about two days.

They still talk about him.

Living Again

I had an awesome weekend with some friends near where I lived during my high school years who I had not seen in ages. We went to the water park, and yes, I wore my bathing suit. All in all, still a good break, but glad to be home. Sort of. Being home meant back to the realities of life and all that entails. Making appointments for my next surgery(ies) and dealing with a cat we were still watching for signs of lingering issues.

Lee also got home this weekend, just after the water park. Of course, I was still angry with him. I always was then. So it was a chilly homecoming. At least he was home, and I didn't have to do everything myself anymore. At least not until the next deployment I reasoned.

I was terrified to start working outside the home, because I have never really worked. I had not worked at a "real job" since I was first married, before kids. I do not know how to organize my time, get shopping done, have time to cook like I love to do, or figure out what was entailed for taking the animals to the vets, or kids to their appointments. At what point to you ask for the time off or just inform the boss that you need to leave?

I finally got the call from social services. The call I had been expecting, dreading, and yet hoping that by getting that call, I could find some peace.

They had found a new adoptive home for my daughter. My part was over. I would be her mom no more. One more meeting to sign the papers was all that was left. I cried for a whole day. I had never cried harder or longer for anything else in my life. Cancer was easy compared to this.

Some tough anniversaries of losses were hitting right now as well. It seems that all the bad things that happen in my life about this time of the year. It was sad, because I love the late summer and early fall with the warm days and cool nights. There was a lot of great weather to be enjoying outside.

I go out to my back deck and listen, and just let the world all go back to the basics of breathe in, breathe out. Sometimes it just seemed like it was so bad that it would never get any better. I knew this was false, and I took comfort in that. At the same time, there would always be **Faith and humor, no matter what.** things going on within the confines of this life. Something was always going to break, someone was always going to get sick, and no matter what, friends and loved ones would die.

It was life.

That does not make it bad, nor does that mean it should not be enjoyed. It just meant it would not be easy. Finding peace in the Lord was about all we could do sometimes. That, and keep your sense of humor. Faith and humor, no matter what.

Monster Waves and Hope

I physically hurt still because of the surgeries, but it was down to more of a constant discomfort, kind of like a little headache that won't go away. Every day I woke up and had to stretch out before I felt better, and I had to do it again every few hours. Someday, I knew I would be better, but it does deplete my reserves of handling difficult situations and difficult people.

I pray and try to read my bible but couldn't seem to find the passages I needed to help my perspective and find the guidance I needed to find my way back into the light. So many who struggle with depression issues understand exactly what this feels like. Many of them lose hope that it would be OK. I had found that as long as you hang on to God, you would be fine.

There is a line in a song that I love. The artists were named Kutless, and the song was "What Faith Could Do." The line was "Hope that doesn't ever end, even when the sky is falling." To me that totally sums up surviving depression: hope.

Hope, for when the sky does seem to be caving in on you, and you are getting attacked from so many places, people, and things. Hope that everything would ultimately be OK, even if that day was not today. Being OK with knowing you may not feel better today or even tomorrow was huge. That was hope, acceptance, and faith.

Sometimes we have no choice but to accept that nothing was within our control, and we are just stuck in these deep waves of emotion trying to merely tread water. The difficult thing to me was the reality that we create some of these monster waves all on our own. They were the actions we took that either didn't go as planned or turned out to be bad choices. Those are the ones that seem to swallow me whole. They are my responsibility, but are now out of my control. How do I fix this? Many times I could not, and there was nothing I could do but try to keep my head above water.

Hope is unbelievably powerful. What would you accomplish if you were not afraid? To me that statement was full of hope. Hope that there was no fear. Hope that you would succeed. Hope that you can handle whatever comes your way. Hope that you would make all the right choices along the way. Hope that the world was a good place and not scary and unsafe all the time. Hope that you could make a difference, and do something good. Hope that your good works would be acknowledged somehow

I learned a valuable lesson along the road I was on: just do the next thing. So I would. The next thing was to take a shower.

Have a good day my friends.

Correction: Have a hopeful day.

Working and Visiting

Amazing things, emotions. They change. One day seems awful, the next you could feel just fine. When you were stressed, (and I was afraid there was still enough going on in my world that I classify as stressed), you learn to really savor the moments when you could just breathe, and let the world whiz by around you while you sit and listen to it all go by.

I was planning on having the final stage of reconstruction done at the same time as having my ovaries and fallopian tubes removed. Well, it seemed as if God had intervened a bit. Due to an insurance snafu, and a scheduling issue between the two doctors, I had to make the choice to either have both done together later (as in running into the holidays) or have just the final reconstruction done in the beginning of October. After much thought and prayer, I decided to separate the two surgeries. I was tired of sleeping on rocks, and I really would like to be comfortable again. The recovery from both surgeries was pretty mild, but the two together would be a bit more. Plus, I was just not yet emotionally prepared to go through menopause. I sort of

274 WHERE'D I PUT MY BOOBS?

was, but I was looking at my life and what I was trying to accomplish at just this moment. If menopause was difficult, I was not willing to risk that yet. In a year, probably, but not right now. Not when I was beginning this new road I was planning to take.

I also didn't want to give anyone the excuse that it was menopause that caused me to divorce Lee. I didn't want to be seen as having acted rashly because of hormonal issues.

Last weekend was awesome. It was busy, and I was fighting a cold, but it was fabulous. One of my big brothers, Earl, the middle of my three brothers, was able to come for a visit before heading to a business trip in a city not too far away for the week. We got to spend some great time together, and he got to see that his little sister had grown up! Yeah, I knew that he knew, but now he really could see it.

We got to go to a small arts festival with a bunch of local artists. One of the artists there was also a breast cancer survivor. She was so sweet; she gave me one of the bracelets she had made. I was so touched that I was sure I was going to cry, and I forgot to pick up her card so I could thank her. Then we went to the second day of the air show that was in town. My brother couldn't even remember the last time he went to an air show. We went to many as kids when my dad was an active-duty Navy pilot, so since he didn't have quite the degree of love for the planes that I do, he had not gone in a long time. It was fun to show him around and discuss all things military.

Passion and Peace

I had come to realize that passion and peace were two very different breeds of cat. I remember praying that I would find what God wanted me to do. I very clearly got an answer. That answer was working with animals, a lifelong love. Yet, every time I tried to work in the field, something happened that stood in my way. I didn't understand it. I thought that this was what He wanted me to do. Why was this hard? Why didn't things just fall into place?

I realize now that I was trying to answer the wrong question. I had asked God what He wanted me to do, and He told me. However, I was asking about what to do for a career, and God was telling me how to be closer to Him.

I was trying to answer the wrong question.

Ultimately, I wanted to be closer to Him in whatever work I did. But what I neglected to realize was that to do the work He would ask of me, I had to be close enough to Him to hear what

He wanted, and not get lost in the noise of what the world (and I) wanted me to do. That was where my first answer came.

The first answer was animals. They gave me a peace I was unable to find anywhere else. See, I have a learning disability. I struggle every day. Doctors tell me it is not ADHD, but it sure mimics it almost perfectly. So I was very distractible, disorganized, and scatterbrained. At the same time, I am able to multitask with the best of them; I can organize better than most when focused and was a great ideas person always thinking of something. The same things that could be seen as deficits were also absolute positive attributes in the right settings. The one thing I had a terrible time doing was slowing down. Everything was in fast forward. I talk fast, write fast, move fast, and think fast.

So, if I was moving so fast, how could I slow down and hear God? That was where the animals came in. One thing about all ADHDer's is the ability to hyper focus ("in the zone") on something that is uniquely theirs. For my son, it was building robots, and Lego® prosthetic limbs, reading, and playing video games. For me, it was working with animals. It was not just interacting with them, but I could just sit and watch them. I could sit and actually sit STILL (ever seen anyone ADHD sit still?) and watch the animal. Here was the thing, for me, I see God in those animals, in the woods, in nature. I could sit, and I could watch, and I could clear my mind, and pray, and be … AT PEACE. Wow! How amazing it was for someone like me who seemed to attract stress, like bees to honey, to find peace. To be able to settle my spirit was wonderful.

OK, so now that I had asked the proper question ("How do I get closer to You, God?") here is the other question that I wanted to ask: "What was Your will for me?" Now, realize, people, that was one loaded question! See, God has this wonderful way of taking you and giving you jobs in His name, that were not at all where you wanted to go. I had heard so many missionaries talk about prayers with God saying "send me anywhere, BUT here..." and they would get sent to "here." Not surprising, after all it causes us to lean upon Him, and depend on Him so that we never forgot why we were doing what we were doing.

This, however, is what ends up becoming our passion when we follow Him. These were things that seem to fall out of the sky, with everything fitting neatly into place with few complications, and it seems that even if you wanted to escape it, it would hunt you down anyhow. For me, it seems, it was my new business. (I would discover later, it was actually writing.) I knew someday I would get cancer. I chose not to work in the field of cancer, or cancer survival, or any of that until now because I had too soft of a heart to hear the stories of those who didn't make it. It was too hard for me to deal with the fact that I would meet these amazing people, only to have to watch some of them die. So, what does God ask me to do? Get involved with support groups for cancer patients and their caregivers, so they could find hope, support, and love, regardless of their diagnosis. I was going to be in contact constantly with people who were hurting and going through more than I had. Some of them would die. I was walking into it gladly, knowing God was there, and also knowing it would be difficult, but so rewarding as well.

My peace was the animals, wildlife, and nature. My passion was helping others find the love and support they need through some of the darkest hours of their lives. God was with me through both. He was in control of both. I just now understand why I need both, and how they are so different. It was as if two more pieces of the puzzle of my life had slipped into place.

I was also rediscovering the other job God had instructed me to do: be a wife. Here I was, upset, angry, "done." He (God) would not let me walk out, even as much as I wanted to. I could not ignore what He wanted me to do. During this time I was also faced with a growing anxiety that I could not put my finger on.

Being Beastly

How do I write about all that was happening when it was all happening so fast? How do I really talk about things when there was so much I was afraid to talk about? I wanted out. I wanted out of this house. I wanted out of his life. I wanted to be on my own. I wanted to find some way to be self-sufficient. I wanted to be OK. I wanted to be done grieving. I didn't know what to do next. All I knew was that I wanted to go. I didn't even know where I wanted to go. I just wanted to go. I was tired of being in a situation where I felt I was being treated disrespectfully. I was tired of feeling like I was being taken advantage of. I was tired of feeling like I had some expectation being put on me about how I was supposed to act even though everything had changed.

I was healing my body, gradually. It had taken a long time, but I was healing. I was not as strong as I once was, but it was coming back. I still had to fight for it, like I've been fighting for everything else. Moving out would be either very helpful, or very painful, or both. I was not sure how it was going to go, but I felt more pressure to move now. I wish I had someplace to go. I knew my options would be larger if I didn't have the animals. They would also be larger if I was willing to move the boys, which I was not. There I go again, still taking care of the other things, putting myself last. I knew that, but I still felt that was my job to put others before myself.

How do I get myself to let go of everyone else, take care of what I want to care for and just be? It would be easier when the boys were out of the house, but now was not that time yet. It was closer. When they were driving and could get jobs of their own, I think that would help. I hated for Alex to feel that he had to get a job soon, but then again, that was just life. I had tried to make it work. I had tried to be compliant, and reasonable. So I thought at the time.

I had tried to accept my "place." It was not working for me. I had stayed thirteen years longer than I had wanted to. That counted for something. I spent years praying about what to do, and how to handle things, even when they never got better. I suffered through my choices alone when I should have had support and love. My stubbornness had caused its own share of problems. Good intentions don't always turn out how we plan.

I was tired. I had tried to be the good little wife, and when the world in which I envisioned living was not working I was told "too bad" rather than "how can we fix this?" I didn't feel that I was considered important enough to change plans for, so I had to change my plans. No major sacrifices were made for me. I went along with whatever was decided for me as often as I could, and that was expected of me. Yet, when I demanded certain sacrifices for myself, I was told I was unreasonable and demanding. I felt I had been treated as if I was not worthy of being treated well. It was always assumed by others that I was being treated well, that he was being treated poorly, that I was always trying to get my own way. Yup, that was why I allowed myself to be dragged all over the world for his job.

Yup, I was unreasonable, and demanding.

I felt as if any move I made would be the wrong one. As if no matter what I did I would be making the wrong choice. How was I supposed to have confidence in myself when I felt as if I had failed at so much? I knew I needed to remind myself of all the things I had done and done well, but they seem so scattered. It's not like I could say I had a great career for fifteen years or something. Thanks to the situation with my daughter, I would never consider myself a successful mom, no matter how good the boys turned out. Yes, I had done neat things for short periods of time, so I knew I could. I just didn't know that I could sustain that. Perhaps by wanting it enough I could sustain it. I didn't know. All I knew was that my dreams were shattered and would never be what I wanted. I had lost faith that those dreams were even possible anymore. Maybe if I would have left thirteen years ago, things would have been better for me. I had a possibility of a fresh start on so many levels. It would have been so hard on the boys. I stayed for them. It would also have been hard on me as well. So I knew on some level I had to admit that I stayed for me.

Now I need to leave for me. But trying to explain that to Alex, not so much Fred, was tough. It all seems so unfair. I was glad my parents waited until I was grown to get divorced, but I did not feel that I could wait anymore. I never wanted to do this to my kids, but then again, what parent does? We all go into things hoping, praying. Sometimes it works, and sometimes it does not.

What I wanted to know was how in the world did they do it in generations past? Were there really just married couples who just dealt with not liking each other and stayed? Were there wives who just sucked it up, and lived unhappily ever after? How did they do it without going insane? How did they do it without hating their husbands? Or did they hate them, but stay anyways? Neither of my grandparents had happy marriages from what I saw. Both sets of them seemed to have very angry, unhappy women with very passive men. That was what I saw from the perspective of a child. I did not have a strong relationship with either of my grandmothers. Both my grandfathers died when I was very young.

By contrast, I saw hubby's grandparents very happy until the end. He doted on her, and cared for her even through Alzheimer's. I wanted that kind of love. I wanted the love that lasted until the dying breaths. I felt that I did not get that at all. But I did have to wonder how my own behavior contributed. I admit that I saw the things he had done to me much more clearly than the things I had done. I also saw all of what I had done to be direct results of what he had done. I had to be acting stubborn here. I had to also have done some of the things wrong to have made this marriage fail. I admit, I sure could not see any of them through the pain. I knew I had been grumpy and unhappy and that had showed, but again, to me they were all direct results of how I was treated. I needed to get perspective. I knew I was a difficult person to live with. I was impulsive, scatterbrained, and yes, I forgot to pay the bills on time sometimes, however, we had never had creditors after us, nor had we ever had anything turned off as a result of that.

I wanted to be OK with the world and my place in it. I always thought my place in this world should be beside my husband. I never felt that is was. I felt as if my place was behind him, shoved out of the way. Now what was my place? I felt like I was eighteen again and had to figure it all out. The problem was I did not feel as optimistic about having the time I needed to figure it out. Nor did I feel I had the amount of options for my life as I did then. At the same time, I had a maturity level now that I did not have then and a very different perspective on life and what was important within it. I was also much more grounded in my faith now than I was then.

In some ways I felt as if I had to explain why I was a good person, even though I knew I was. I was harshly judged by others who never bothered to look deeper than the end of their own noses. I found myself becoming more and more judgmental as well, and that was not a trait I liked to possess. I had become very judgmental in regards to some of the very issues I had been wrongfully judged myself. Not cool.

At some level a part of me did not care. "Judge not lest ye be judged." I've been judged, now it was my turn, thank you very much...

Of course that was totally wrong, but I wondered if there was a part of me that was rationalizing my own judgmental attitude because of that. I was always on guard, always ready to defend myself at every turn, and I felt that I had to do it alone.

My marriage had become so dark in my sight that nothing he did was worth noting or mentioning. He vacuumed the other day. I leave that to him, as I hate vacuuming. I'm sure he expected me to notice and say thanks, but I didn't. I didn't feel like it was worth mentioning, just like I didn't expect him to thank me for doing the dishes or shopping. It's my job. He should not have to be constantly thanked for doing his job. The problem with this scenario was that he thinks the vacuuming was my job, and I should thank him for doing my job. He thought he was trying, he really did. He was more compliant, and helped out more around the house (like I felt he should have been doing all along), but it didn't matter. It felt like a menial last ditch effort to show me that he was trying. There was so much more he could be doing to show me he was trying, but he wasn't doing much more than I would expect him to do. It was not like his efforts were noteworthy.

I sure had on a thick pair of blinders, didn't I?

I knew that my own attitude was not in the right place. At the same time, I really just couldn't see where or how I needed to change it. When he made choices that hurt me, I reacted, but then I was a bad person for reacting in the way I did. I had an issue with that. Mainly: What right does he think he has to treat me that way in the first place? Why couldn't I react how it made me feel? Why must I be denied my emotions and reactions? Why was it OK to be treated wrongfully, but not OK to react in righteous anger? I had to change my behavior? Why didn't he have to change his? If I was reacting, why does the change process have to start with me? Why shouldn't it change with the source? I was concentrating too much on what I felt his job was, and not concentrating on what mine was.

I knew that I was not seeing things clearly. I knew that I was not giving him credit where it was deserved. And I knew now how much I discounted everything he did for me during my cancer surgeries and infections.

This was important to add because of how much can change during cancer with our relationships. So many women have to endure being abandoned, divorced, walked out on, told they were hideous, and all sorts of horrible things. On my front, Lee did everything right, was wonderfully supportive, and I was the one being beastly.

We need to be willing to admit our failings, no matter how bad. It doesn't make us bad people, it makes us human. We are all human, we all make mistakes, and we should all own our own mistakes, and be open to learning how to fix them.

M.A.D.

I had a stark realization not too long ago. I was getting feeling back on my arm! It has been so gradual that I didn't even know it until I was shaving and realized that there were spots I could feel that had been numb. Healing was a wonderful thing! Just goes to prove that it doesn't happen overnight.

I think I was regaining some form of feeling in my breasts as well. Although I still could not feel temperatures or light touch, I could feel pressure, and it finally didn't hurt anymore. The sensation was a bit bizarre, but not painful anymore. It would be interesting to see what comes back as time passes.

My final reconstruction surgery was scheduled for 06 October 2010. It would be outpatient, performed right there in the doctor's office. It would take longer to sew me up than it would to remove the expanders and place the implants. I had been told by others who had been down this path that the recovery was a piece of cake. I admit I was skeptical at this moment only because of all the problems I had with the secondary infection the first time around. However, I did feel more empowered to do my part to keep that from recurring and to have a quick and boring recovery. I would be using a surgical scrub all over when I take my shower the day of surgery. Every little bit helps. Gee, I better be sure to get every speck of fur off all my clothes that day too. That may be too challenging. After all, no outfit was complete without a little cat hair!

I was still adjusting to my new size. Forget shape for now as that would be different after surgery, which was good since I was still lumpy and lopsided. I was realizing that my clothes fit differently and that I would have to adjust what I thought fit. I used to pick sizes in shirts based on how they fit across the back. I never had to make an adjustment based on the front. I think perhaps there was some wicked conspiracy between clothing manufacturers that they should base the way their clothes fit off of the assumption that everyone was a C or D cup size. I say this because my shirts do seem to suddenly actually fit as if they were intended to, and I did not have all this extra room in the front anymore. I never did any tailoring to my clothes and looking at how they fit now, I was realizing I had been walking around for years with droopy shirts.

My plan for my new life was starting to take shape, slowly but surely. I was trying not to run without looking where I was going. Part of me was totally stressed about it, and part of me was so excited that I want to jump right in and got it moving. I love it because I finally felt as if I was going to make a difference.

Making a difference…Making A Difference: M.A.D.

That was a new movement: Be a M.A.D. woman! I like it that I was beginning to feel that I was becoming a M.A.D. woman. I had already been accused of a bit of that, but now I could really fulfill that one. Sounds good to me!

Note to self: Be strong, be courageous, be a M.A.D. woman!

Realities

One of the things that happen in the reconstruction process was the rebuilding of the nipple and areolas. This was done by taking some skin from your back (yeah, more scars), and fashioning a circular shape along with the creation of a nipple and sewing it to the front of each breast in the appropriate place.

These were the last of the surgeries, and only the tattooing of the nipple and areolas were left after that. I made the choice to forego those two procedures. One might wonder why. The main reason that I got reconstruction was so I could look good and normal in my clothes. I didn't want to have to worry about my prosthetics falling out if I bent over, wearing a bathing suit, the costs of prosthetics or bras, etc. But as I sat alone in the dark on my back porch this morning, I realized I was not quite being honest with myself about it all. There was more to this decision that the looks aspect.

I had to really dig deep to explore what that was, and I was surprised at what I found. As you may have noticed, I had not had too much trouble dealing with the cancer and all that was thrown at me. I acknowledge that I was "disfigured" and that the scars would always be there. I knew that this was the beginning of my road, and I was OK with that. However…

I found a place inside of me where there was some significant grief that I politely chose to ignore. The role the old breasts played in my sexuality. This was a difficult topic to address, but the purpose of writing all of this was to let you all come on this journey with me. This was definitely part of that journey.

> There was some significant grief that I politely chose to ignore.

As you know, breasts play a very important role in our sexuality. Men go gaga over them. They watch the breasts instead of the face when the topic of conversation is boring. They watch them go up and down during exercise and notice every woman not wearing a proper bra, or none at all. Men's minds think in sexual connotations. That was reality. When dating, the breasts were "second base." It was an achievement in the progression of the dating process.

One of the starkest memories I had was "second base" with my hubby. I could actually remember what I was wearing those twenty years ago, and the fact that that pale yellow tank top had a pink spot near the shoulder where I had spilled food or beverage of some kind on it at one point. I remember where we were, and even how the clothes felt. My shorts were a little bit tight, not too much, but I noticed—he probably did too.

As life progresses, and relationships too, the breasts play a big role in the comforting and nurturing of not only our spouse or significant others, but our children. I didn't know of any women out there who didn't love to have their special ones lay their heads on our chests, on our "pillows," and what a comfort that feels to us as well. There was something womanly complete about someone laying their head on your chest and just resting.

That was gone. That role, all of it, was gone. It would not be replaced if I got a fake nipple. The sensations, from the emotional biochemical reactions to anything dealing with the breasts were just GONE.

I found that terribly sad. It was a sadness I had not yet faced because I didn't want to. I didn't want to accept that reality, that loss. The loss of looks does not bother me. But the loss of the sensations tied to those nipples had been horrible to lose. They played such a vital role in my sexuality, and they were no more. It affects my libido. It affects if, how or whether I want to be touched at all.

Something as silly as "how could you tell if I was cold?" actually has a sting of pain. I joke about it anyhow. It gets me through. The nerves still react, or did for a while, and it was a bizarre sensation, feeling my body attempt to contract the no longer existent nipples, and then give up and go away.

Why reconstruct the nipples if their total function was gone? Why bother? I realized I had this silly recurring fear that in the heat of the moment, one of the nipples would be inadvertently twisted off, or sucked off, whatever. How silly, I know. And how gruesome. But the underlying issue was that no matter what, I would not feel it. I could blissfully laugh it off and go "oh, look at that!" but I would not feel a thing. That pain that I would not feel was something that I would miss as much as the pleasant sensations associated with them. I didn't want fake ones there anymore only as a sad reminder of their lack of function. How that part of me would never feel again.

I would not miss the "deer in the headlights" look that caused me to forever wear thick, heavily padded bras, and I felt as if I was trying to make myself look that way, when I didn't want to look perpetually cold. I could now wear thin bras that were light and comfortable, if I want to wear one at all. That was a plus. Adding reconstructed nipples would return the "deer." That I did not need. I felt different enough being a bit bigger now than I was.

So I sat and cried a little about it, and felt a bit silly for doing so. But it was still a loss for me and needed to be grieved. I heard a great quote that perks me up at times like that "yes, they were fake, my real ones tried to kill me!" There was so much truth, sad truth, to that. But I was here, most of me, and I was doing OK. I could open the window and enjoy the beautiful day God has created. I could continue to enjoy my life, and all its trials and tribulations.

There were harder things to grieve than those two pink spots. I need to learn to grieve the loss of friends.

Five of us at church were diagnosed with cancer within two weeks, four of us on that second week. I was the only one under sixty-five. That was in January. As of today, only two of us are still alive. I found that I could not go to their funerals. I had done so much crying on my own, I did not want to do more crying in public. No one else needed to see it for now. After all, I should be grateful. I was going to be OK. It seemed like a slam to show up when I was OK, and they were gone.

Life always goes on. I take great comfort in that; the continuity of life. I look at the clouds, the trees, and I feel the wind. I know they would all be here no matter what. It was almost fall, and the leaves would turn, and again I would get to feel the crunch beneath my feet. The walnuts on my trees had begun to fall (thanks to the squirrels), and I hear thunking sounds as they drop onto my rooftop. Again, it would snow and get cold. Later it would warm and flowers would grow and birds would sing. Then it would get hot and the fireflies and the cicada would return as well. Of this I could be certain; I would be cleaning up after the occasional yakking cat. I'm grateful that even though I do not know who would be with me, God and all His creation most assuredly would be.

And that, dear friends, was enough.

Adjustments

Did I tell you I graduated from physical therapy? I did, I did! What a wonderful feeling. If I didn't have my next surgery still ahead, I would almost feel like all of this was finally over. I had a great last day of PT on Friday. I really worked it. I was lifting weights beyond what I had been working with since before surgery. I was sure sore afterward, but it was the good sore. I love it. Then I went to the gym yesterday. I wore my hot pick breast cancer shirt that says "Save the Ta-tas." You can tell who reads it because they get this little smirk on their faces as they walk past me. I needed to get the companion shirt that then says, "Caught you looking!"

So, I go over the benches to work with my oh so impressive three-pound free weights. The guy sitting at bench next to me was not really sure what to think of me sitting next to him. I was straining to lift a flippin' three-pound weight, when he's sitting there all muscle bound with a seventy-five-pound weight in each hand. I felt somewhat stupid, but I hoped he'd be able to figure it out by the shirt. Then again; he was a guy, true. Maybe that meant he was really distracted by my implants instead. I was not sure which was better or worse.

How I would adjust to a "work schedule," since I had not ever really had one? I sat down and figured up how much time I had been spending working on things. It was just little bits here and there throughout the day. I realized I was putting in about 6 hours without even trying! I guess that was what they mean by if you enjoy your job you don't even notice you are working.

Since writing this counts as "writing a book," I was including the time I spent writing, too. The nice thing about doing this from home was that I could start work when I woke up, so if I was just plain up at o'dark thirty, I could get to work and really crank out my day. I was still trying to get a handle on organizing doctors and vet appointments. I realize everyone has to make these adjustments, but when you've never had to before, it could be a little intimidating. Then again, I did not have a boss who I had to ask for time off. I worried about making mistakes that impacted others when I worked outside the home.

Everyone makes mistakes in their lives. We pick ourselves up, fix it (or just leave it), and then move on, and hopefully we learned the lesson in the process. I look back at a lot of the things I made mistakes on, and I realized that I had done OK.

Then I look ahead and take a deep breath. I would not borrow trouble, I knew God was with me, and I would do fine.

I was looking forward to doing the Susan G. Komen Race for the Cure on the 03 October 2010. That would also be just days before my final implant surgery. I hoped to meet a ton of fascinating women and men who were all banding together in hope for a cure.

Because You Were My Friend

Two of the most important things you can do for another person with whom you were emotionally connected were to (a) Give them a hug, and (b) Tell them you love them. I know that most guys will not go for this, thinking it is not masculine and all. That was true in my sons' cases. However, let's get past the stigmas and down to brass tacks here. These two important things cause very important physiological reactions.

I read somewhere that people who are hugged more have less depression. It is the same with people who are told they are loved. The reason, I believe, is that when someone tells you they love you, you know that you are loved, which is a basic human need. Hugging releases endorphins and dopamine, which are hormones that help our bodies feel better (I read that somewhere, but do not remember where ... so don't ask). The same thing happens when someone we care about says they love us. They promote healing in the mind, body and spirit.

I had started making it an especially important point to hug my single girlfriends and tell them I loved them. I tell my married girl friends as well, but I knew that many of my single friends did not get that as much as they needed. Then again, neither do some of my married girlfriends.

People who are hugged more have less depression.

Of course it takes on a totally different meaning if I were to say that to a guy. I had noticed (via Facebook) that there were some guys who had taken to doing this very thing and had found an amusing way to express themselves without giving the wrong impression: "Non-homo love you bro." While this is not politically correct by any means, it gets the point across that you are my friend, and I love you for being my friend.

How cool is that?

Those kinds of sentiments and actions make a huge difference in people's lives: Especially when things are tough. Especially when you are feeling low. Especially when you are sick. Especially when you feel alone.

I pondered the proper protocol of this very subject and how it applies to the opposite sex. Obviously, if I tell any of my male friends that I love them, it would be a whole different ball game (ignore the pun, please). They deserve to be told they were loved as well, but it was not appropriate. It made me wonder if the above statement ("Non-homo love you bro") could somehow be adapted to fit the guys in my life. I'll be taking suggestions.

Times when you feel so alone, no matter what the reason, having someone tell you they love you is a reaffirmation that life is good because you are loved. I had no idea how many people thought of me until I got cancer. I got tons of cards and was totally blown away. When I was feeling low I looked at them and reminded myself that the person who sent me this card cared enough about me to send it. I was loved, even if from a distance.

Most people who are suicidal will tell you that no one cares about them, yet for so many of them, their funerals are packed with people who do love them. Tell people you love them and value them. Tell people they mean something to you. Give them a hug.

In the meantime, consider yourself hugged, and know that I love you because you are my friend.

And yet, I foolishly left my husband completely out of this scenario, out of anger, for many more months yet to come.

My Toy Box

I saw a post yesterday on my favorite Facebook page, Beyond the Boobie Trap, which really got me thinking. The post was basically this: "Was there a day that went by that you forgot you had cancer?" I thought I would answer that in regards to myself.

The answer, as of today, was no. No, there was not a moment that went by that I forgot. Then again, I was still in the process. Things still feel weird. I was still healing, recovering, and getting used to my body again. I was still regaining strength, stamina, and even regaining some feeling in areas that I had written off as numb. I still had another surgery ahead to finish the job. That would be in just a few weeks from now.

That being said, I was not letting it define who I was, but I was letting it motivate me to live a better life. I try to be kinder to those who seem grumpy. I found that I was proud of myself for having chosen to live a "stop and smell the roses" kind of life in the first place, so I really didn't feel that I was missing much. I was, however, starting to try to do more for myself, rather than putting myself last. This was easier as my boys were getting older and did not need me as much. I was redefining my dreams, and what that meant. I was trying to embrace peace within myself and find calm. I was more set on finding ways to help others.

My faith did not take a beating through all this. Many people do go through a time where they were mad at God or question why. I did not have that, but that was my walk. My faith has always been rock solid in that department. That was just me. I think hanging onto that faith was very important to help you get through. To be able to accept that someone else was in control when you had none, and that it would all work out for good in the end was huge. Hang on to that. It helps in the dark, painful hours. Think of being forged iron. How does iron get strong? It gets its strength by being heated to the temperature of Hades and then beaten with a hammer until it was the right shape, then drenched in cold water. Sound fun? Nope, but that's how iron gets strong.

I was through trying to make every relationship or friendship work if it really wasn't meant to work. If I had to work too hard to stay in that person's favor, it was not worth it. I had incredible friends and family, who I felt I had neglected, and they had been with me through so much. They were enough. I decided they were more important to hold on to than to spend my efforts trying to make difficult relationships work. Besides, I got so much more joy out of seeing them than the dread of "was this going to be a good time or a struggle?" with the difficult relationships. I do not need the stress. I had enough of that, thank you.

I was getting past the need to make everyone around me happy or to have everyone like me. I did the best I could in my own quirky, ADHD-type way, and that was good enough. Not everyone could handle me. Then again, I could not handle everyone, either. There were some people who just rubbed me the wrong way. It didn't mean they were not a good person. I just could not connect with them on their level. Some people could not connect with me on mine, and that was alright. It's life, it's me, and that is OK.

When you get cancer, everything changes. Everything. It's like someone took the bucket of toys that was your life and dumped it all out into the trash. Now you were trying to sift through the garbage to try and save your favorite toys from that bucket and learn to leave the ones that were not so important anymore or leave the ones that were just plain broken. Along the way, you discover new toys to embrace and enjoy. Find which toys are important to you, and take them out and play with them. Don't put them in some box under the bed, in the closet, or in the attic. Enjoy them while they last. They will not last forever, and even in you live to be one hundred, you will not live forever, either.

"If you live to be 100, I hope I live to be 100 minus one day, so I never have to live without you." – *Winnie the Pooh.*

Underwire Nightmares

The countdown was really on. On 06 October 2010 I would get the permanent new pair. I was dreaming of how much more comfortable they would be. I was wishing for nights I could comfortably sleep on my side and stomach. I was dreaming of nice fitting shirts and dresses.

I had a picture taken of me recently, and I didn't recognize myself at first glance. My figure has really changed. I was amazed at how different I look to myself. I was told by Lee that I "posture" when I walk past the mirror. If I do, it's totally unintentional, but I still look different. It was a change. It would be another change when the final ones were in. I'll be glad to be less lumpy looking as well. Shirts fit differently. I had to re-evaluate what constitutes a shirt fitting or being too tight. I put on button down shirts and go "NO!" as the buttons gap. They always seemed to gap for me, now they really gap. It is an easy fix by wearing a camisole. They still fit through the back. Just differently, so I'm adjusting.

Another noteworthy thing: underwire bras. I could not wear them. I could not wear them for now, simply because

I was placed too far apart, and the cups do not reach that far out. Add to that, the underwires hit right at the scars that were left by the tubes, and they really hurt. I mention this because I went into Victoria's Secret the other day, and some cute young sales gal in her mid-20s was trying to convince me to try on their "new underwire" that was supposedly a bit more padded than the old ones. I tried to tell her I could not, and she persisted that they were SO much more comfortable.

This was probably the first time since surgery that I really wanted to smack someone for not listening about mastectomies. I realize it was the sales pitch, but it really ticked me off. It hurt that I was ignored when I said they would hurt. This gal had no clue how bad they would hurt, and I was angry that she didn't change tactics and show me bras that had no underwire.

I had never been as tempted to talk to the manager as I was that moment. I didn't only because I didn't want to embarrass the gal, because I realized she had no clue about what I was experiencing. I did see this as a potential learning opportunity for the store, and I may go in and talk to them. They lose a lot of customers like me with that kind of attitude.

The statistics I had seen say that someone was diagnosed with breast cancer every minute or less, depending on what you read. That was a huge demographic of women who may be needing softer bras. Perhaps the store's demographic was only younger, "whole" women. It might be worth it to ask that question.

I felt as if my journey with all this was almost over, even though I still had to take care of the ovaries. That part would have challenges of its own, but they would be very different from the ones I was experiencing now. Having the ovaries taken out would not directly change my appearance. I may have a weight change (hopefully not too much!), but I would not go through the dramatic changes I was undergoing right now. There was a bit of relief in that. Relief in knowing that some surgeries do not leave the scars that this one has.

Race for the Cure

It was a bright, crisp, "frost on the pumpkin" type of morning. The sun was rising steadily by the time I got to the area I was parking. I put on three layers of clothes so as to avoid a heavy coat and to be able to peel off a layer if it actually got warm enough, or if I actually worked up a sweat. I met briefly with the group I signed up under, but not really knowing anyone I quickly lost them all in the crowds.

I joined the thousands of other participants for the race as we made our way to the Civic Auditorium in Omaha. Each turn of a corner added more and more people. It was a sea of pink by the time I reached my destination.

My first stop was to find the registration table: I needed to get the right shirt. I had on one that was white, but because I was a cancer veteran, I got a pink one. I felt special. I was given a pink shirt, a pink hat, and a pink racer's number. I proceeded to get the tags where you put who you were racing for.

I promptly and completely went blank. I had been thinking about the list of people I planned on putting on there, but the names decided to play hide and seek in my memory. So I put down who I could think of off the top of my head (that made it a short list). It included my mother and my two aunts for "in honor of." Then I put Delynn, who was a neighbor of mine, and Carol, our church matriarch, for "in memory of." Then I put the tags on my back with a little help from one of the other racers.

I wandered around a bit, watched all the people. What a day to take a brisk walk with about 19,000 of my closest friends. As I watched the people milling around and then gather for the first race, the one-mile, I was amazed at the number of supporters. I saw plenty of cancer veterans, but I was very thrilled to see so many supporters of cancer veterans there. I saw many teams that were there in honor of one person, often someone who was with them. I saw whole families walking for their mothers, grandmothers, aunts, sisters, etc.

Then the one-mile race started. I felt like I was in NYC watching something there, because I had never seen the likes of it here in Nebraska. All the people; this solid looking, undulate mass of people, all happily walking down the street.

And then I thought of more names to add... Jane, Bev, and Genae, and all the gals at the Beyond The Boobie Trap online.

Then came our turn; the three-mile race. I realized I had not walked that far in ages. I was having so much fun watching this equally large mass that I was now a part of, pour down the streets in front of me like a wave of pink

Kool-Aid. The line of people spread out the entire three miles. At the front were the runners and the line was solid from the beginning runner to the ending walker.

Spirits were lifted, voices filled with joy, laughter in the air. If I hadn't known any better, I would have thought this was some kind of revival.

People everywhere were discussing life, survival, memories, faith, and hope, all for each other. All in the hope that in our efforts, we could find a cure and keep our sisters, and our daughters, and our friends from ever having to go through this.

The teams had names: Mammary Militia, Pink Soldiers, So-and-so's Team. They had themes, usually pink (imagine that!). I had never seen so many men unabashedly wearing pink as on that walk. There were lots of slogans as well: Big and small love them all! Save the Boobies! Feel your Boobs! All reminding us to get mammograms, support the cause, etc.

I was inspired to see so many other cancer veterans. I was fascinated to see how many were so lovingly supported by family and friends. I knew how much that meant to me to be surrounded by those people. It was fabulous to see that support at the race. I underestimated how that would affect me, and I regretted deeply that I did not ask for people to walk with me.

I should have. I needed that, but did not realize that I would. Next year would be different. Next year I would have my own race team. Next year, maybe, just maybe, there would be a cure. Maybe next year, we would not need to race. Maybe, next year we could cure cancer.

The New Me

Well, yet again I look in the mirror and do not recognize the boobs in front of me. Part of this was because of the obvious swelling from surgery, and part of it was because the shape was quite different than I was expecting. The easiest way to describe this was less projection, more circumference. I made sure to recheck all the paperwork to make sure he put in the right size and shape. I had faith that he had, but I looked so different from what I thought I would, that I had to make sure.

These implants were high profile. That meant that they were narrower, and stuck out more than the other types. This surprised me now that they were in, because they did not seem to project nearly as much as the expanders did. It all seemed a bit odd that everything looked so different than I was expecting. Now, I realize that there was still swelling going on, but I had no idea how much. I had heard different stories from different people in regards to this. Many stated that there really was not much swelling, and that what you see was a pretty good idea of what you now had.

I was grateful he used a type of buried suture, and no tape. That would really save me as far as more rashes from adhesives. I already had an itchy spot just where they had the monitors stuck on me during surgery. The suture line he used was so smooth, that I could not even see it. The only evidence I had of them (prior to reduced swelling) were the two blue threads sticking out of either end or the suture line, indicating a start and stop point. Awesome!

True to form, he and I continued to joke about sizes even up until the final surgery. He walked in and asked if I was ready for my 900 milliliters. I unblinkingly said "yes!" and my poor hubby did a momentary double take wondering what he had missed. Of course I got the 600 milliliters, and that was definitely enough. I think the less projection would be good in the long run as I would not be banging into doors and people as much.

No drain tubes, very little pain; this was all good. I was on pain meds, but really not much. The skin was numb per previous surgeries, so no pain there. My body did react to the trauma anyhow by just feeling a bit sluggish and achy, but that was to be expected. I did have on a compression bra to help with the swelling. I was not sure how long I would be wearing that. I had a follow-up on Monday to have a look at everything. Today was Saturday, day three after surgery.

The doctor was right, the silicone was definitely more "normal" feeling. I'm not sure how much of what I was feeling right now was swelling as opposed to implant, but they do squish similar to what the normal ones used to.

They do not bounce anymore, but we knew that. I could not feel the edges of the implants, like I could with the expanders, but part of that may be swelling as well.

I could once again cross my arms in front of me. I missed that silly, simple gesture. Being constantly cold, I cross my arms a lot, so being unable to do that through the majority of this year had been awkward. Now, I could give myself a hug again.

The medication was telling me that it was yet again time to lie down before I fell down, even though I was already sitting. It would be nice to get off of the pain meds again, but it was not quite time yet. I said continued prayers for a boring recovery, and I was hoping to move around enough to wake up the bowels but not enough to exhaust myself.

Good days ahead.

Lee was there for me every step of the way. Driving me to and from surgery and follow-up appointments. He was always telling me I looked beautiful. And then he would go to work, and I would spend hours looking on the computer for someplace to live. I still hadn't realized that I was already living in denial. I had already moved there, and set up a home, and been living there for quite a while. The state of denial is a lonely and dark place. I do not recommend moving there any time soon.

Fluffing the Pillows

I had my follow up appointment with my plastic surgeon yesterday. My progress has been wonderfully, blessedly, easy thus far, and I could not be more grateful. Handling the meds and all their side effects was a breeze since I had so much practice earlier this year. I knew exactly what to look for on my scars, and what coloration was normal.

The doctor was pleased with my progress and he removed the stitches. As I mentioned, all you could see were two threads on either side of the incision, and that was it. This type of suture was called a subcuticular uninterrupted suture. Basically, think of a simple sewing stitch where you just go back and forth in the material. This kind of stitch was similar to that. Consequently, taking out the stitches was amusingly easy. You simply pull one of the suture threads firmly but gently, and the whole thread slides right on out. This way, you do not see any scars caused by the stitches. I imagine this stitch was some of the life blood of the plastic surgeons' repertoire for reconstruction.

The stitches were out, and then I suddenly felt like I was being sent to the movies in an obscure version of the movie, Roxanne, with Steve Martin.

"Now, you have to massage these new implants a lot for a while, and really get them to move around so they keep the more normal feel and movement and get them to sit in the right place in your chest." The doctor said.

Excuse me? Did he just tell me I needed to have my pillows fluffed up?

Why, yes. Yes he did.

Of course, the smile that crossed my husband's face as he quickly started saying "they're doctor's orders, now," was to be expected. As amusing as that was to be hearing, I was waiting for the hidden cameras to pop out to catalog my startled reaction.

Those were definitely the most obscure doctor's orders I had ever received. I knew my husband would be very happy to carry those out to the letter as well.

I remember, sitting in that doctor's office and hearing the instructions. I waited until the doc had left the room, and I pointedly looked at Lee, glaringly, and said "Didn't get too excited about this. I don't plan on letting you or anyone else follow those orders to the letter."

Boy, I was a stubborn pill, wasn't I?

I found it amusing that I had to use a lot of ice on my new pair for the first forty-eight hours post-surgery. You see, I hate the cold with a passion. Telling me to use ice was the one thing I would absolutely be a noncompliant patient about. I could not stand it, except in this case.

The beauty of this situation was that I needed to ice what was already permanently numb from the first set of surgeries. It's not hard to ice what you could not feel anyhow. Well, that was cool.

No pun intended.

Works for me. So I made sure I had the proper amount of layering between the ice and myself so that I did not cause ice burns, and I iced away. There was a lot of swelling, so being tolerant of the ice was a good thing.

My scars really do not look much different than they did before this last surgery. It's funny because without those typical sutures, and the fact that these were removed so soon afterward, I kind of felt like I was going to pop them back open.

I was talking to my recently widowed brother, Rich, about the doctor's orders and we had a good laugh when he mentioned that as a trained care-giver, perhaps he could make a living massaging the implants of women who didn't have someone to do it for them. He could even wear a blindfold for those for those who were shy. I told him to camp out at the local plastic surgeons' office. He might just get some takers.

Then I had a bit of a laugh to myself thinking that it would be so funny if that actually happened, and if he started dating one of the women. Can you imagine the story?

"So, how did you two meet?"

It could happen.

Lessons

Seeing as how I was off of all medications and in virtually no pain with only slight discomfort, I could sleep again and had no more surgeries ahead for my cancer, (save the ovary removal), I guess this would be my last update.

I discovered that Victoria's Secret was, from now on, going to be safe with her. I would not need it. There was a part of me that was a little disappointed. Wouldn't we all love to be able to look as good in our undies as they portray that we would? I walked through the store yesterday and discovered there was nothing that I wanted to wear. Nothing was going to be comfortable. Perhaps it was a sign of age, perhaps maturity. Either way, I was good.

My goal in my journey has been to find some semblance of a normal appearance with my clothes on while out in public. I believed that I had now achieved that, thanks in great part to my plastic surgeon. Out of clothes, the evidence was obvious that the pair I now sport was not at all real. That's OK. My surgeries and illness could fade back into the background of my life. It would always be at the forefront of my mind, but I hope it remains in the background of my life, at least for a time.

It was time for me to move onward and upward, and to do new and better things. There was a lot of work ahead for me, and that was OK. I hope to make some good progress and ultimately make a difference for someone else. This was my goal.

As expected, cancer has rearranged my life. It has strengthened it, and given it direction and purpose. I am thankful that my faith never wavered, nor did any of you. I want to thank you all so much for being on this journey with me. It meant the world. So much of the battle with cancer is a lonely road that only other cancer veterans can understand, but that doesn't mean we don't want or desperately need everyone else to surround us with their love and support. You all have done that for me. I cannot thank you enough. There are stories of terminal cancer patients fighting back, and winning, due in part of the support, love, and attitude they had. Then there are stories of cancer patients with the best prognosis who died, because they simply lacked the will to fight and loved ones to surround them.

So I feel confident in saying to all of you: thank you for saving my life. I mean that to each and every one of you who so much as thought "I hope she is OK." It mattered. It matters to all of us.

Thank you for saving my life.

- Take away from my story these things:
- Be kinder than necessary. Everyone is fighting some kind of battle.
- Be the change you wish to see in the world.
- Keep your sense of humor no matter what. There is humor in everything if you only look for it.
- Ask yourself what you would do if you knew you could not fail.
- There is no failure, only the failure to try.
- Live and love with all you have.
- Find both your peace and your passion.
- Never let go of God.
- Tell your family and friends you love them .Someday it will be the last time you get that chance.

Thank you. I love you all. Come back and visit anytime. My door is always open and the coffee is always available. Just remember to ignore the dirt. I cleaned a few days ago, so sorry you missed it. If I didn't get up to greet you at the door, it means I must have a cat or two on my lap, so just come on in and make yourself at home.

Learning to Listen

As with life, the story didn't really end there. God had other plans. He always does, doesn't he?

There seems to be an underestimated stage of cancer recovery that I was unaware of, even as recently as the time of the last note. I had spoken to several people, and pretty much across the board, no matter what kind of cancer or treatment, it has been the same.

Once treatment was finished, you would think that it would be a time of great joy and basically it was. Yet at the same time, this ugly specter raises its being and engulfs us in a rather unexpected act. Suddenly, when we should be celebrating, and glad, and rejoicing, all we wanted to do was climb into some dark hole, and not come out.

Depression and anxiety hit like a tornado. I had previously thought (as had many others) that this was just a function of the chemotherapy, radiation, and all the other hormonal things that happen to our bodies during the trauma of cancer. Not necessarily so. I also thought that this was an indication of the fear of reoccurrence of the cancer, which like the first time around, really didn't scare me.

So I was totally blindsided by this new battle to fight. I had not had any radical treatments, save for my surgeries. I had not had my ovaries destroyed or yanked out (yet). I was not terrified of it coming back; I expected it. So when I started to feel absolutely exhausted, could not sleep hardly at all, which had nothing to do with comfort, and started feeling this tightness in my chest all the time, I was confused. I was sure the mono was recurring, but the test showed I was fine.

Hmm. OK. Great.

Now I was at a place where I was ready to start "taking on the world" as a veteran, and I could barely function enough to spend an hour working or getting dinner made. How fair was that? I wanted to be done and OK again. The end of treatment should mark that, but it did not. It was merely a marker of the beginning of a new road with different things to deal with.

Welcome to the new normal.

Some people find this stage easier than others. For some, a good bit of prayer and rest help and then they are fine. Others plummet into a pit of despair from which they feel there was no return. I was somewhere in the middle. I do not yet know if I would need medication for this. If you do, by all means get it! These depressions and anxiety issues are hormonally based, and the concept of thinking your way out of a true depression or anxiety issue was like willing yourself to fly; you can't. You can't control your hormones.

You can control your thoughts though. That was why I was trying to figure it all out. My thoughts were right where they should be. I had no fear of recurrence; I did not feel hopeless, helpless, or otherwise. I did, however, feel this as yet unnamed fear in my chest that would not go away.

I found a house about this time that I could afford, and it had everything I needed and wanted to start anew. I was filling out the paperwork, and it hit me like a punch in the chest, the tightness. The anxiety picked that exact moment to hit, and I was paralyzed. I could not fill out another line. I could not even think about moving without spinning out of control and feeling like my chest was being squeezed in half. I know now that it was my subconscious telling me that under no uncertain terms was I ready to move out just yet. That things between my husband and me were not over, even if I wanted them to be.

That was the beginning of really listening. Listening to my body, to Lee, to the other veterans and what they were going through in their own relationships. The door I thought I had nailed shut was once again coming unlocked and light was beginning to shine through. A new place was on the other side of that door. A place I was not expecting. I was about to peer through and decide I actually liked what I found. Life with Lee could be safe and good after all. I discovered I could put my life in his hands and not only was he trustworthy, but capable and

Your life may never be the same, but it might be even better.

loving, even if I didn't want to acknowledge it. I also discovered that I did still love him, in spite of my anger. I found out most of all that all of this was good.

I would be going to find a counselor to help with the anxiety. Many patients who go through this get medications from their oncologists. I would certainly bring this up to him. It feels like a slap in the face to have to deal with yet another health issue that was out of my control. At least this one was not life threatening to me. It was for many others, so get help if you need it.

I found great comfort in talking to all my friends, both cancer veterans and those who had not had to face this. Each one brings a new perspective. Communicate with them and your family. Sometimes you feel alone simply because you did not tell anyone what you needed.

I read a "Dear Abby" type column, where this gal had a mastectomy and that was it. She had an easy recovery, physically, but felt no one acknowledged her pain and loss. She probably didn't ask for any. Or perhaps those she turned to could not understand, and she just did not know where to go.

Find other survivors who do understand. Sometimes they are the only ones who can. There are resources out there to help you do that. There is the American Cancer Society, LiveStrong, and Susan G. Komen for starters. Find help. Find support. Communicate with your friends and family and allow them to help you!

Allow them to help you fix dinner one night. Allow them to help you clean your house. Allow them to help you drive to doctors' appointments.

You are a veteran! Be proud of that, but accept help when you need it; there is no shame in that. Let them pray for you and with you. This is a long hard road. No one should have to walk it alone. I am here. I am with you. I can empathize.

I am a veteran, too.

Made in the USA
Charleston, SC
13 November 2012